I0102533

THE
ESSENE
DIET

THE ESSENE DIET

THE HOLISTIC PATHWAY TO HEALTH AND WEIGHT LOSS

Dr. John Hagan

Rauson Group LLC

Copyright © 2013

John Hagan, M.D. Rauson Group LLC

ISBN 978-0-9820828-2-9

LCCN 2012953044

Contact: dietstudy@gmx.com
2313 L-S #138, San Antonio, Texas 78230
Psychology consultant Nels Oas, PhD
Proofreading courtesy of Mary Jackson

Table of Contents

Graphics and Tables

Introduction

The Essenes were a mystical sect of Jewish priests that existed for over 500 years before being lost to history early in the Christian Era.

They lived communally in dedicated houses in small towns and villages in ancient Judea and Galilee. Though priests, the men took pride in working as craftsmen, shepherds, or common laborers in their communities.

The Essenes were known as the healthiest men of their time with many living past the century mark. They ate simple foods and were not vegetarians. Significantly, their first meal of the day was taken after a morning of work.

The Essene approach to diet forms the basis for this book. The ancients knew that a daily morning fast helped lay the foundation for mental, spiritual, and physical health. For the obese of our own time, it can result in weight loss.

Chapter 1 The Essene Diet

...(the Essenes)...are long-lived also, insomuch that many of them live above a hundred years, by means of the simplicity of their diet; nay, as I think, by means of the regular course of life they observe also. (Josephus, *Wars of the Jews;* book II, chapter 8)

Whether the Essene morning fast ritual came about through divine revelation or from simple observation of what made them the healthiest, it served them well for hundreds of years. Can the morning fast concept have a relevancy in modern times?

The human species has not changed appreciably in 20,000 years, so the benefits the Essenes enjoyed should hold true for us today.   To study this question, a modification of the Essene daily fast was developed and tested by a group of volunteers in a pilot study.

The 14-10 "track" is at the core of the adaption. The fast period runs for 14 hours and the "free" period for the next 10 hours. For the person on a normal schedule, the fast begins at 9 p.m., continuing on through the night and ending at 11 a.m. the next morning. During it, only the drinking of water is allowed. In contrast, for the following 10 hours, there are absolutely no restrictions on the type and amount of food eaten. This is termed the "free" period.

At first look, the protocol seems to fly in the face of logic. How can weight be lost with unlimited food intake? A lot of food can be eaten in 10 hours! Worse, breakfast needs to be skipped completely, and isn't breakfast the most important meal of the day?

But the results in our study volunteers were positive — and even surprising. So before dismissing the approach out of hand, take time to read the real-life experiences of several participants in the Essene Diet program, written in their own words.

Terri

I am a 34 yr old female. I am married with one 10 year old son. I have been overweight most of my life. I have tried many ways to lose weight. I have been semi-successful on the LA Weight loss program, and being a vegetarian and working out 5 days a week at the gym during college. Then I got down to about 160lbs. But alas those were many years ago and I am back to just over 200lbs.

Terri's actual weight was 208 pounds. After she learned about physiology and the rationale behind the program, she became enthused. Previously, she thought it was important to eat breakfast and never missed it. Terri started the protocol the day after the first meeting. In a week, she reported back.

I have been not eating from about 9pm till noon the next day. I have found that during my noon meal if I eat more protein, I don't feel hungry the rest of the day, including the need to graze. Also the hunger I feel kind of turns off in the morning now.

The rules are that there are no restrictions on what you eat. Terri took advantage of it, as we read in future communications.

Today was an off day due to a pot luck at work. Yesterday was tough. For some reason the BBQ chicken and Mac n cheese during the student's lunch had me salivating. I have been eating what I like, trying to increase the fruit a bit as I know it's good for me. But I have had Taco Bell and Wendy's this week, as well as homemade food like a BLT, nacho's, shrimp Alfredo with veggie's. I will hop on the scale sat morning before coming to..(the meeting).. to see how it's going.

Terri was keeping to the protocol as best she could, but she also had a busy life.

I have been sticking to the protocol mostly. During camping with my son I did have a bite to eat in the morning. I have not been losing much weight though. I thought maybe it was due to my menses, but that is done for the month now. I will stick with it the rest of this week and see what Saturday shows. I have been very thirsty, and not very hungry during the morning. I have been tracking all the food I eat just to see the calories in vs calories out with the walking I am doing. But my pants seem bigger?? So I am not sure what is going on.

One month after starting the Essene Diet, this is what she had to say.

I am doing well. I pulled on jeans the other day fresh out of the dryer (when they are the smallest) and they were really loose! I was very excited. My stomach is shrinking. I can only eat about 3/4 of what I would eat before. I am bringing home leftovers from restaurants on a regular basis. My cravings change, too. Some days its for chocolate and peanut butter. Other days its guacamole and veggies. But I eat what I like.

Six weeks out, this was her report.

I had a major AHH moment. I went bridesmaid dress shopping on Sunday. I usually am a size 20 in a normal store. The lady at the store said the dresses run small by 2 sizes, so off to try on a 22/24. OH MY GOODNESS, it was HUGE! And not just a little big. I had to go to a size 18. Also tried on some 16 pants, and I could get them on and buttoned, still tight but huge progress. So something is definitely happening to my body.

I am continuing to take walks with the dog and my stomach has gotten very small. I am not able to eat as much as before so I am making better choices. I have found when I eat more nutritionally dense foods I am not hungry. If I eat junk I get cravings. So more fruits and veggies for me.

After seven weeks, Terri reported a weight of 192 pounds, down from her initial weight of 208 — all this without any food restrictions or requirements for exercise.

Terri reported that she thought her stomach was shrinking because she couldn't eat as much as usual. And her food cravings were changing for the better.

As weeks turned into months without a report, I thought Terri had been "lost to follow-up." But then I received an email from her seven months after the last communication. She had been through a lot emotionally and had strayed off the protocol several times, but always came back to it.

..to date I am down to 180lbs, from about 208!!!...Have not felt like I have dieted a single day...I can do this forever!

Denny

Denny is a 39 year old man with a life-long weight problem. As he writes:

I'm not on any medications and my health is excellent other than the fact I am overweight. I've tried some fad diets over the years... Adkins diet with some success but, it didn't get me the full results I wanted and then when I went off the diet I was worse off then when I started it. Last year I changed to an all healthy food diet while on a regular work out regiment, which produced the best and steadiest results I have ever had. Now I know how to lose the weight, but, need my mind set to change. While growing up, all of my family was very healthy other than my father who was always eating snacks...While growing up I was the only kid out of 5 that ate like food was going out of style. I was adopted when I turned 5, but, that's really the only unique thing that happened when I was a kid. I had a great upbringing and I have a fantastic home life now.

Denny, too, was convinced by the physiology and began the protocol. Two weeks out, he reported back:

Everything is going great! I have only eaten a couple times in the early morning because we were guests somewhere and I usually will eat if my host prepares something. Other than that it has been relatively easy to stick to the plan. My cravings for sweets has tapered significantly. Both my roommate and I have noticed that we both get full much more easily at meals... We've noticed more of a change over the last week.

Four weeks into the program, Denny was noticing more changes.

We eat less and are more satisfied. No more late night cravings before bed. We are both sleeping better and feel rested in the morning when we wake up. I have cheated some mornings around 9:30am or later and forget that I am supposed to wait until after 11:30. I have lost approximately 7 pounds. The greatest thing about this has been my loss of severe cravings for sugar or fatty foods. I still want them from time to time, but, it's much easier to control the cravings.

Most curious. Denny's cravings for sugar or fatty foods have been blunted. He doesn't eat as much as before and is sleeping better. And Denny is losing weight.
All this as a result of a morning fast?

Don

My name is Don. I am 39 years old. I am divorced with no children. I am 5'8'', 240 lbs.
I was heavy in high school. Between 1991 and 1997, I joined college ROTC where I lost weight running about a mile a day and became somewhat bulimic for that summer to lose weight for the uniform. Lost enough weight to earn the uniform, but left the ROTC program and then regained weight.
In 2000, I did LA weight loss and lost 30-40 lbs, down to 180. I joined the Marines few months later. I kept weight off in Marines by exercising and running 5 miles a day. I got married in 2003 and slowly gained weight. I left the Marines in 2004 and over time gained weight to put me at 225. In 2010 did a low carb diet similar to Akins and lost about 30lbs. But I divorced later that year and gained the weight back.
Currently I am at 240 lbs and have started a portion control diet this week, and have lost 3 lbs on it..
My health is good. I have had my appendix taken out, and in the last year I have had slightly high blood pressure, for which I am currently taking Lisinopril at 10mg. I was on an anxiety medication, but have had a sleep study done and now I have a CPAP machine. It has improved my mood and getting restful sleep.
Family history: Parents are both alive. I have one brother and one sister. They are both still married with children. My family is heavyset on both sides, but otherwise in relatively good health.

After a little over two weeks, Don was finding positive results.

> My hunger pangs are gone. I have lost around 4 pounds (but see it flux a little). I weigh myself at the same time everyday. I am drinking lots of water and drink soda very little. I don't have the craving for sweets and alcohol as much...I am feeling better and find myself doing more things around the house. Sundays I have a hard time sticking to the fasting period because I get up around 7am and go to bed around noon.

Don is getting used to what he previously thought was hunger. He doesn't feel urge to eat just because he knows is stomach is becoming empty. Amazingly, Don has lost his craving for sweets — and alcohol. And he is losing weight.

Scott

Scott, age 50, is married with a son and enjoys lifting weights — a life-long discipline with him.

Scott wasn't even close to being overweight, much less being obese. He wanted, however, to squeeze off another 10-15 pounds in order to get down to what he thought his ideal weight should be.

After the initial contact by email and learning it was a behavior-based program, Scott thought it would not work for him.

> I am sorry to say, but at this point I am probably not going to be a good subject since I noticed your study centers on behavior-modification as opposed to a new diet technique.

> I used to be 320 pounds and was pre-diabetic (along with many other weight related problems). I now am 185 and have

had normal blood glucose for over 2 years... No more weight related medical problems of any kind.

I was able to change due to behavior modification. I simply made changes in my life that I knew I could live with the rest of my life and that were helpful in my goal to lose weight.

I have about 15-20 pounds to lose, but have tried for over a year without success. My Dr. says that he believes my body will genetically not allow me to lose any more weight. Short of starvation (which I refuse to ever do again), I have tried every diet that any doctor, dietician or fitness trainer has to offer.
So as you can see, I would not work well with your study.

Scott had an keen interest in exercise and physiology, so I suggested he come to one of the meetings just for the information.

Scott agreed. After hearing the logic behind the Essene Diet, he decided to give it a try. He continued with his morning weight training workouts during the fast period.

Scott reported after the first week.

..Otherwise, yesterday progress was good and today I did my first workout at 5:30 (cardio and weights) -- had my first bite to eat at 11:30.

The results were surprising. Usually I am famished, but my body is getting used to eating later. Also my thirst was high enough that I kept drinking water and never got hunger pains.
I am also going to attempt to cut off eating at 7PM in the evening so that when possible, I will be fasting for 16 hours before I eat. (7PM to 11 AM typically)

Three weeks into the protocol, Scott emailed me with a teaser.

> I will give you a long update in the next week or two - not until I have more data and am absolutely assured things are on the right track.
>
> But if things continue for the next couple weeks (and I don't see why they won't) , all I can say is **WOW ! ! !**

Two weeks later, I received the report. As I suspected, the weight loss was minimal because Scott was in great shape to begin with. But Scott found other benefits that surprised me.

> Now I will say, even though my scale weight has not been great, there is one <u>consistent</u> thing I have found about not eating breakfast. When I was a teenager and used to lift weights, I would be sore the next day, lightly sore the following, and basically recovered after 3 days. Before I started your program, I would not get very sore the following day of a workout (delayed), on the 2nd day I would be bloody sore, and it would often last for 3-7 days. Considering I have been lifting for almost 2 years now come January, my soreness was not due to untrained muscles. Now that I have started skipping breakfast and working out first thing in the morning, my soreness pattern has reverted back to the *same pattern as when I was a teenager*. This has been a very consistent pattern.
> I have also noticed a few other consistent changes:
>
> * I used to have ravenous cravings for food after a heavy workout. Now the cravings are slight to non-existent.
> * It is easier to keep my caloric intake to (what I want)
> * I am less moody than I used to be when I cut calories.

Scott also noted that he is gaining strength.

> I still can't get over the change in soreness and how fast I recover now. I feels surreal and the amounts I am able to lift have steadily increased. For example, my bench went from 135 1 rep max to 155. I can now do 135 eight times.

> Also, I have not changed any workout techniques or supplements. The one and only change was delaying my first meal of the day.

Scott's results were totally unexpected. Why was he getting stronger with exercise, and with an improved recovery time as well?

Many of the following chapters deal with human physiology in an attempt to discover an explanation for what Scott and others reported. The bare-bones science information is intentionally presented at a college level out of respect for the reader—who should at least have an appreciation for how complex human physiology really is. The internet is a good resource for further information on topics of interest. The reference I used is the professional standard on the subject—Guyton's Textbook of Medical Physiology, 12th edition.

Along with physiology, chapters also deal with cultural issues such as the failure of commercial diet programs and the development of the "cult" of breakfast. Also, the reader will be taken on a trip into the ancient world of the Essenes and learn about other approaches to diet and fasting.

But perhaps you—a healthy overweight adult—have already been convinced by our study participants. If so, the program can be easily started today. At some point, however, please make an effort to read the rest of the book. Making health decisions based on testimonials alone is never a good idea.

Chapter 2 The Myth of Breakfast

It is a cultural myth that the eating of breakfast is essential for good health in an adult. This belief was created by a powerful breakfast food industry and helped along by well-meaning but over-solicitous parents. Worse, for overweight adults seeking to lose weight, making breakfast a part of their routine virtually assures long-term failure.

> You've probably heard "breakfast is the most important meal of the day" enough times that you've started to tune out – but it's true. When you think about it, there's usually 8–12 hours between dinner the night before and breakfast, so it's the first chance you get to refuel. Breakfast can also help kick-start your metabolism. (Kellogg's "Love Your Cereal" website Sept 2012)

Kellogg's cannot be faulted for promoting their breakfast food business, however the above paragraph is simply not accurate — based on what we know about human physiology and metabolics.

Cereal giant Kellogg's is not alone in playing fast and loose with science. Ads pushing the importance of breakfast are everywhere. A fast-food chain recently centered a national advertising campaign on "arresting" people for skipping breakfast. "Got to get the metabolic machinery!" is a popular and unchallenged catchphrase breezily tossed off by TV pitchmen and nutritional "experts" alike in the justification for breakfast.

Thinking of the human body as the biological equivalent of an internal combustion engine is a common popular misconception which is exploited by the breakfast food industry. Outwardly, the analogy seems logical. A car needs gasoline in order to run, and a human being needs food in order to live. Ergo, in the morning, the stomach needs to be filled with food for the day ahead, much like filling up an empty gas tank in a car before taking it out on a long road trip. How can one function on an empty stomach?!

But how our bodies break down food for energy is vastly more complicated than the workings of any gasoline-powered engine. Furthermore, nothing about our basic metabolism needs to be "started up" in the morning by food. And as for the human stomach serving as a fuel tank, well, that is true only in a very general sense.

Six fuel Tanks, Not Just One

The engine analogy, as faulty as it is, is useful and we will stick with it to illustrate how things really work. True, the human body has only one food "tank," the stomach. But the food has to be processed extensively before it can be turned into the body's equivalent of gasoline. In fact, to be properly compared to an engine, the human body must be allowed not one but six fuel tanks, with many more "sub" tanks possible depending upon how finely the biochemistry is parsed.

Let us explore the nature of these six energy reservoirs. For convention, "HT" will stand for "Human Tank" and will be followed by a number from 1-6.

HT1 is indeed the stomach, and it includes the small intestine as well. Here, the food is initially stored and then slowly digested and broken down into three basic nutritional elements which are passed on into the body through various mechanisms. Each of these basic elements we will now give their own symbolic tank.

HT2 holds the breakdown products of carbohydrates (sugars and starches). The carbohydrates absorbed are processed in the liver and re-released into the bloodstream as 95% glucose. Once in the individual cells of the body, most of the glucose that is not immediately needed is polymerized into storage granules called glycogen.

HT3 holds lipids (fats). Most of these fats reside in adipose tissue as neutral triglycerides and some in the liver. This fuel tank must be reduced in size if weight is to be lost! For the average male, HT3 amounts to 15% of his weight. In females, level is 24%.

HT4 holds amino acids and the protein made from them. Amino acids are used as fuel only as a last resort. For the individual who is not starving, HT4 is not a major factor in fueling the body. This tank includes muscle tissue, enzymes, hormones, and other types of proteins.

These basic substances can be biochemically transformed into one another in the liver depending upon the immediate needs of the body, with the exception of a few amino acids. Most importantly, both HT2 and HT4 have limits. If more carbohydrates or protein are ingested than can be stored, the excess is converted to fat and placed in HT3.

The Real Fuel Tank

Now for the fuel tank of the body which is directly analogous to the car's gasoline tank. We will call it HT5. It is filled with a substance called adenosine tri-phosphate, or ATP. It is from this tank that the body draws the energy to drive the metabolic reactions that take place within the body's cells.

The car engine derives its energy from the explosive breaking of the carbon-hydrogen (C-H) bonds in gasoline. The human body also derives its energy from the breaking of C-H bonds, but those that are found in the molecules of carbohydrates, fats, and protein.

In the cell, through a complex series of coupled reactions, the biologic C-H bond energy is transformed, or transferred, into the phosphate-oxygen (P-O) bonds of the ATP molecule. Each ATP molecule in HT5 has two such bonds—gained from the breakdown of either glucose (HT2), fatty acids (HT3), or amino acids (HT4).

To complete our metabolic model, HT5 is connected to a separate tank, HT6. When HT5 is full of ATP, the excess is chemically transformed into the high-energy molecule phosphocreatine and stored in HT6. The reservoir of energy in HT6 is drawn upon by HT5 when the body's needs are immediate and ATP is being burned rapidly. The phosphocreatine in HT6 can be broken down in seconds for ATP, where ATP production from HT2 and HT3 takes a minute or more to ramp up. As an example, in athletics, sprinters and weightlifters depend on the energy stored in HT6, phosphocreatine, for their power.

Putting it All Together

Scientists now have a good idea how the fuel in these six tanks is used over time and under specific conditions. Normally, HT5 will first draw fuel from HT2 (carbohydrates) to replenish its store of ATP. When the fuel in HT2 is low, HT5 will then shift over and access HT3 (fats) for the needed ATP. Finally, and as a last resort, HT5 will

Human Energy "Tanks"

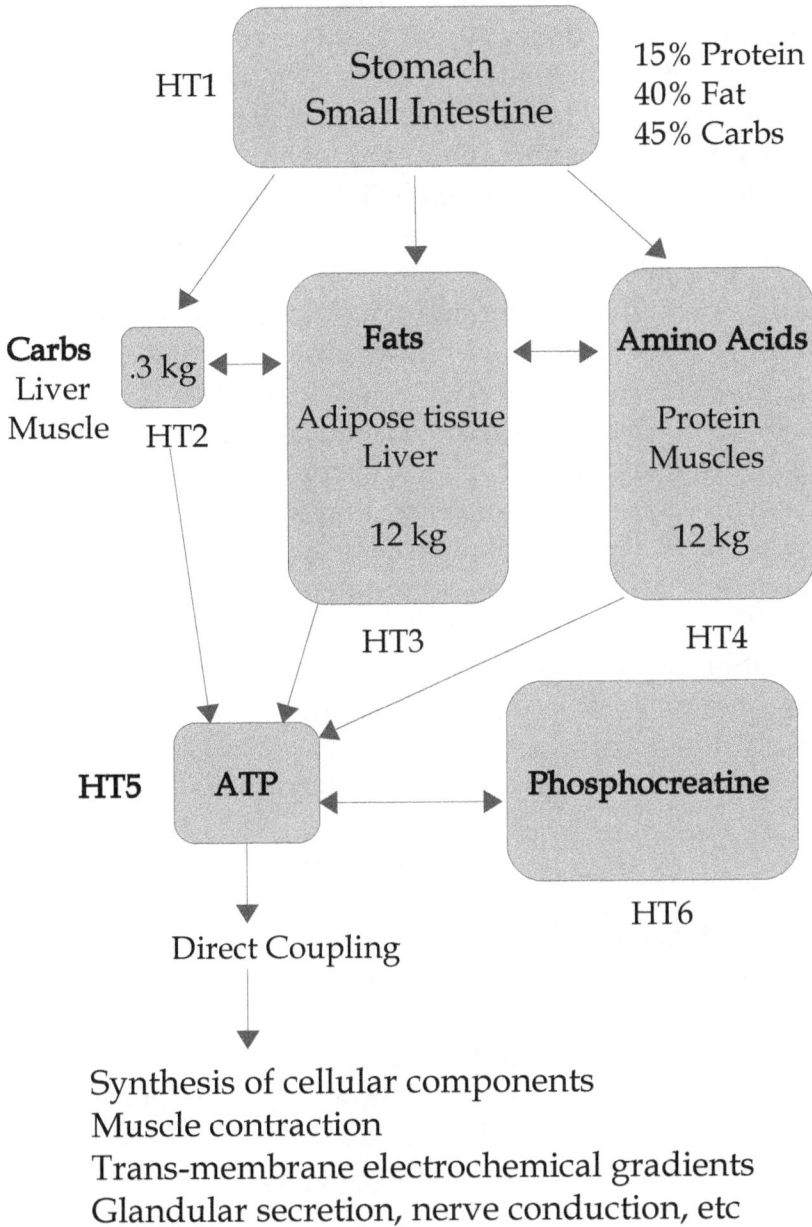

Stomach
Small Intestine

HT1

15% Protein
40% Fat
45% Carbs

Carbs
Liver
Muscle

.3 kg

HT2

Fats

Adipose tissue
Liver

12 kg

HT3

Amino Acids

Protein
Muscles

12 kg

HT4

HT5   ATP

Phosphocreatine

HT6

Direct Coupling

Synthesis of cellular components
Muscle contraction
Trans-membrane electrochemical gradients
Glandular secretion, nerve conduction, etc

turn to HT4 (amino acids) for fuel. For emergency bursts of energy, HT6 (phosphocreatine) is drawn upon.

In the morning after a night of fasting, the stomach (HT1) is indeed empty, but now we know that HT1 is simply a holding tank, a "pre-fuel" tank, if you will—as are HT2, HT3, and HT4. The real fuel tank of the body, HT5, has remained full the entire time you slept. During the night, the body's complex biochemical processes functioned as they needed to without missing a beat, and with all the ATP fuel they required.

Additionally, a key finding by researchers is this: In the morning, HT5 has shifted away from being replenished from the burning of carbohydrates in HT2 to the burning fats in HT3. This is of great consequence for the dieter and will be discussed further in later chapters.

Many people have concerns that in the morning their glucose level will fall dangerously low without breakfast. That fear, however, is unfounded. The human body regulates serum glucose very tightly. In the morning, while the rest of the body is burning fats, the serum glucose is still being maintained adequately. Stored glycogen is being broken down for glucose, and, if the glycogen levels are low, glucose is being synthesized from amino acids.

Take Home Points

The body's metabolism does NOT need to be kick-started in the morning by eating corn flakes or any other food.

In the healthy adult, the serum glucose is kept at normal levels even if breakfast is not eaten.

As an extreme example of how well the body stores energy, a well-nourished individual can fast and remain alive for several weeks—as long as water is available to drink.

Chapter 3 Hunger Set-Points

All men are born weight-appropriate, yet everywhere there is obesity.
                                                                    -*after* Rousseau

"If breakfast is not essential, then why am I hungry when I wake up in the morning?"

A good and logical question. What, exactly, is the nature of hunger? And why, to some, is the urge to eat difficult to resist?

The origin of the sensation of hunger is complex. A strong influence is the continuous stream of messages that the brain receives concerning the state of the stomach and the level of blood nutrients—glucose, fats, and amino acids. Psychology, however, is also a major factor, and will be the focus of this chapter.

As we have just learned, the body has plenty of stored pre-fuel from which to make ATP—several weeks' worth, in fact. Most of the time the stomach should be empty. But for most, the association of an empty stomach with the need for food is strong and difficult to break. In the obese, an empty stomach usually does not remain empty for long!

But we all know people who skip meals and are not concerned about it. Usually, these people do not have a weight problem. Do they have a unique and enviable set of genes, or is there a behavior-based psychological reason for their apparent control over hunger?

Stomach Physiology

The stomach is composed of involuntary "smooth" muscle. This type of muscle has an intrinsic electrical rhythm, which, if strong enough, causes a contraction to occur. The contraction then moves through the stomach in a slow and coordinated fashion. A single contraction of smooth muscle can last for hours. This is in contrast to striated or skeletal muscle, where contractions are under volitional control. There, the response is immediate and powerful, but relatively short-lived.

Stomach muscle contractions can also begin reflexively when food enters the stomach and stretches its smooth muscle walls. These circumferential contractions start in the mid-body of the stomach and occur every 15-20 seconds. They move in slow waves towards the pylorus, gaining force as they do so. The pylorus is a small muscle-ringed orifice that connects the stomach with the small intestine.

When the slow primary contractions get close enough to the pylorus, the pylorus smooth musculature is stimulated to generate its own rhythmic counter-waves. These contractions push the food back towards the body of the stomach. As the strength of the pyloric contractions diminish, the the primary contractions again dominate and the food material is pushed back towards the pylorus. This is repeated and over and over, resulting in a churning action.

At the same time, the gastric glands lining a part of the stomach endothelium begin to secrete mucous and digestive enzymes. The stomach's parietal cells also secrete hydrochloric acid. The mixing of the food contents with the digestive enzymes and acidic mucous produces a substance called chyme. Bit by bit the chyme is pushed through the pylorus and into the small intestine.

The Fasting Stomach

Contractions, however, can also begin on their own when there is no food in the stomach — usually after the stomach has been empty for several hours. These are called hunger contractions and also originate in the mid-portion of the stomach. These contractions can "fuse" and cause a continuing tonic contraction that can last for 2-3 minutes.

The fasting contractions are most intense in young people, whose muscle tone is usually very high. These contractions also occur when the blood sugar is low-normal. A person experiencing them might feel mild pain in the pit of their stomach — called a hunger pang. These pangs do not begin until 12-24 hours after food was last ingested. They reach their peak over 3-4 days with continued fasting, after which the pangs gradually weaken.

Interestingly, a similar discomfort pattern has been reported by some on the Essene Diet morning fast protocol. This is despite the fact that the fast is only for a few hours, and the participants are free to eat as much as they want for the rest of the day. The intensity of their morning hunger and stomach pangs tended to peak in four days and then diminish — as if they had been fasting the entire time.

Evolutionary Instincts

The human body evolved from primitive organisms over hundreds of millions of years. During that time, a strong built-in neural bias developed towards food consumption. Those organisms that were able to extract, store, and utilize energy in the most efficient manner were more likely to survive and so reproduce — passing on their genome to following generations.

It is clear that there are powerful internal mechanisms in place to drive the human body to get the nutrition that it needs. Studies have consistently shown that toddlers and pre-school children will, over time, eat a balanced diet if left to their own devices, and a variety of food is presented to them.

As an extreme example, a pregnant woman can develop the Pica syndrome, in which she has a strong urge to eat dirt or clay. Many will act on this urge. But the outwardly irrational act is driven by a very rational purpose — to obtain iron to make hemoglobin for her and her developing fetus. The body somehow knows what it wants.

In both situations, the sense of smell — with its three distinct evolutionary layers — likely plays a dominant role. However, the take-home lesson should not be that we are slaves to our hunger impulses, but rather that the brain has its own circuitry for food acquisition that, when necessary, can override learned behavior.

Given that obesity is driven by hunger, the question must be asked: does obesity serve a rational evolutionary purpose, or is obesity an aberrant physiologic development unique to our times of abundance?

Negative long-term health issues with the obese suggests the latter. There are also other anti-evolutionary aspects to obesity — social, hygienic, basic mobility considerations, etc — that would tend to lower the chances of the obese finding a mate and successfully reproducing (though some would argue that point!).

For these reasons, a major assumption of the Essene Diet is that obesity is not a natural outcome of evolution, but rather a corruption of it. It is further postulated that external factors in modern life tend to disrupt the body's natural set-points — with aberrant hunger impulses being just one of them.

The Physiology of Psychology

Scientists are discovering that psychological conditioning has a physiologic basis which can be observed under brain microscopy. The brain itself gains information through billions of sensory neurons throughout the body. Most of this information is screened out ("habituated") and never reaches the level of consciousness—having been adjudged to be superfluous and so "locked" out of the brain. This prevents memory storage overload.

The human central nervous system in total is composed of 100 billion neurons. Neurons can transmit messages of an "on-off" nature down their length—lengths which in some cases can be measured in feet. Each of these 100 billion neurons has between 1,000 and 200,000 interconnections with other neurons. These are called "synapses" and can serve a variety of functions.

A synaptic connection can be of several types. A synapse can serve to either passively transmit a signal from one neuron to another or modify the signal in transmission either positively or negatively. The two primary neurons can themselves be modified through synaptic connections with other neurons, those neurons can have their own modifying neurons, and the iterations can continue on to astounding levels of complexity. This is the essence of a neural network.

Brain Plasticity

As infants grow, the number of neurons and synaptic connections grow as well. In infancy and into adolescence, there is a pruning process of these neuronal connections based on the "use or lose it" concept.

While the study of memory in humans is difficult, studies in primitive animals have been revealing. Short-term memory is associated with chemical changes in the involved neural pathway synapses. Through repetition, the short-term memory can be "consolidated" into long-term memory. This process involves DNA-driven protein synthesis — resulting in changes which can be seen microscopically. This makes the memory "file" — which is actually a complex network with connections to many parts of the brain — readily accessible.

When these primitive organisms are given a drug that blocks the DNA stimulation of protein synthesis, these short-term memory patterns will not be consolidated, and permanent memory is not made. This explains the retrograde amnesia that some humans experience after a convulsion or a severe concussion; the memories preceding the traumatic event for several minutes are completely lost. Why? The traumatic event interrupted the brain's consolidation process.

This also indicates that human synaptic networks physically change over time depending on the changing stimuli they are exposed to. The plastic quality of all neural networks is important to appreciate. In large measure, this explains how the human animal learns, adapts, and changes old habits — which are well-proven concepts from psychology.

The brain controls behavior, certainly. But now we know that changing behavior — i.e. repeatedly and consistently changing the stimulus patterns the brain is exposed to — can also physically change the brain.

Normalizing the Set Points

Many outside factors in today's world play to the hunger urge—which by evolutionary design is easy to trigger. Consumption of breakfast upon awakening, for example, could be a ritual learned as a child and carried over into adulthood. Or it could result from psychological osmosis from decades of exposure to breakfast food commercials, with the perception of hunger being a secondary factor. The field of advertising is very sophisticated. Subtle cues are carefully placed in media ads to encourage consumption whether food is needed or not.

For those seeking to lose weight, the brain's neural plasticity can work in their favor. By consistently resisting the urge to eat, as one has do daily in the morning fast protocol, the brain circuitry begins to rewire. Appetite and satiety set-points that have been corrupted over the years begin to normalize. Over time, the neurological connections linking the urge to eat with the sensation of an empty stomach becomes either attenuated or superseded by new circuitry. As our test participants uniformly reported, on the fast protocol, over time, the sensation of hunger becomes blunted, and the cravings for specific "bad" foods either diminish or disappear altogether.

Other physiologic set-points might also be effected by this fast-induced renormalization process, including mood and "addiction" disorders. More research is needed in this area.

The popular aphorism "you are what you eat" has been largely debunked in the previous chapter. Most all foodstuffs we consume are broken down into very basic elements which can then be converted into one another under the right conditions. But what is becoming more and more apparent is that the aphorism "you are what you do" is a very true statement and strongly rooted in brain physiology.

Take Home Points

The human animal will instinctively seek out the food that it needs for optimal physiologic functioning. This is likely driven by man's sense of smell.

The evolutionary urge to eat when food is available, but not really needed, has been reinforced —corrupted! —by today's pro-consumption, media- driven culture.

The brain's neural circuitry is plastic and can be rewired. While the brain controls behavior, changing behavior can also physically modify the brain —over time.

Chapter 4 Commercial Diet Programs

Nationally advertised commercial diet programs are numerous and make implied promises to those seeking to lose weight. However, the long term results for these approaches are so dismal that no program reports their results fully—if they bother to track them at all. The FTC now requires advertisements for commercial programs and dietary supplements to disclose real-life expectations. Most often this results in a disclaimer that the results reported — usually spectacular—are not "typical."

This is an understatement.

In 2007, a revealing study out of UCLA was published.

Mann T, Tomiyama A,; *Medicare's Search for Effective Obesity Treatments: Diets Are Not the Answer* ; April 2007 American Psychologist

As its title suggests, Mann *et al* found that with diet-only programs any short-term weight loss is regained over the next five years. The diet programs only differ in the rate of regain—the most "successful" of them having the longest rebound time. Even more damning, the UCLA researchers found that individuals who are obese but with a stable weight are better off health-wise than the obese who intermittently lose weight through dieting and gain it back.

The data analyzed was so convincing that the authors concluded it was pointless to even study the question any longer.

..there is little support for the notion that diets lead to lasting weight loss or health benefits.

Is dieting a threat to public health?!

Perhaps in response to this, commercial diet programs now add an exercise "kicker" to their recommended protocols. In fact, most programs recommend an intensive enough exercise program that even without dieting the individual will lose weight. This begs the question: if people can lose weight through exercise alone, then why go on a diet?

Most commercial weight loss programs have web sites. Let us look at two of the most heavily advertised, Weight Watchers and Jenny Craig.

Weight Watchers

Weight Watchers (WW) is one of the oldest commercial plans available. Calories are restricted by assigning foods and portion sizes a number value and limiting the number of points that can be consumed in a day. No foods are absolutely forbidden, but the high-calorie foods are given a correspondingly high point value.

The program, along with counseling and encouragement, is available online. Also, from their internet web site it is easy to join a local group where a personal counselor is assigned to each participant, and weekly supportive meetings are held.

There is a modest disclaimer on the web site (Sept 2012). Amid the impressive testimonials is a sentence which states that participants who follow the Weight Watchers plan can expect to lose 1-2 pounds per week.

But how many of those who join follow the program for any length of time? What is the drop-out rate? No data is given.

Deeper in the web site is a "terms and conditions" section. Item 14, in small print, is a another disclaimer.

This Website provides weight loss management and information applications and content published over the Internet and is intended only to assist users in their personal weight loss efforts.

There is no promise or guarantee of results, just of assistance in the participant's "personal" weight loss efforts. But that is certainly understandable because eating is a totally volitional act.

More disingenuous is the WW "consumer bill of rights," also deep in the web site. The first article of the bill:

The Weight Watchers weight loss plan is designed for a safe rate of weight loss - up to two pounds per week (after the first three weeks). If you lose at a greater rate, you must review the Plan guidelines and adapt them, if necessary, to avoid rapid weight loss. Not following the Plan as designed may pose the risk of developing health complications associated with rapid weight loss.

Thanks for the heads-up! It is reassuring to know that WW's number one concern is people who lose weight too quickly on their program.

In article two of the "bill of rights" lies the real disclaimer.

Only permanent lifestyle changes - such as making healthful food choices and increasing physical activity - promote long-term weight loss.

Increasing physical activity. Eating less. Of course. If you did that, you might not even need WW!

To their credit, WW has at least attempted follow-up studies on their own participants. One study in particular is of interest.

Lowe M, Miller-Kovach K; *Weight-loss maintenance in overweight individuals one to five years following successful completion of a commercial weight loss program;* March 2001 International Journal of Obesity.

The study was initiated in response to the 1992 NIH Technology Assessment Task Force report. The NIH report found that on average as little as one-third of the weight that was lost in the participants in these largely academic-based studies was kept off after one year, and none of it after five years.

This was not good news to Weight Watchers.

First author Lowe put together a study in cooperation with Weight Watchers because of concerns that the patient populations referenced in the NIH report did not reflect real world people—such as those individuals who might join Weight Watchers.

Fair enough. But those whom Lowe and colleagues chose to study out of the pool of Weight Watchers' participants was also selective. It included only the success stories of WW—"Lifetime" members—, those who had maintained their target weight loss goal (5-10% of their starting weight) for six weeks. But even among that elite group, those who had a 30 and over BMI—the truly obese "success" stories—

were omitted. Lifetime members followed were in the overweight category with a BMI between 25-30.

BMI stands for body mass index. It is determined by dividing an individual's weight in kilograms by the square of their height in meters. It is not a perfect measure of weight status. Muscular people tend to have a higher BMI than they rightfully deserve, but it has become the reference standard none-the-less.

In this select WW group, the follow-up results were admittedly significantly better than those reported in the NIH report. Adjusted for error inherent in self-reported data, the study found that after two years, participants maintained 72% of their weight loss. After five years, participants maintained an average of 50% of their initial weight loss.

But how many people who joined Weight Watchers failed to hit their goal weight or dropped out early? Weight Watchers doesn't say. And concerning those Lifetime members with a BMI over 30? Sorry — not included.

Looking at the big picture, it should be kept in mind that WW sets the bar very low in defining a successful participant. A five-percent weight loss in a 200-pound person is 10 pounds, which would only drop them from 200 to 190 pounds. For a female who is 5'9", to drop from 200 pounds to 190 pounds represents a BMI drop of 30 to 28.5. Compare this to the accepted standard weight for a woman of that height of 146 pounds or a 22 BMI. While statistically there are health benefits to even this small of a weight loss, to call it a success is, at the very least, disingenuous.

A better question for WW to consider is this: How many people achieve their IDEAL weight through their program? How many 200-pound people get down to even 160 pounds and keep it off five years out?

Jenny Craig

Jenny Craig (JC) sells meals and snacks that can be bought at a JC center or home-delivered for a fee. JC also offers online or local group support counseling.

The JC website opens to an introductory page where a toll free number is listed to call for more information. Conveniently, there is also a form that can be filled out and emailed from within the site to have a representative call you.

Clicking about to the different pages, amidst the slew of testimonials from attractive people, there can be found hard data on the program. The average individual who joins JC can expect to lose 1-2 pounds per week. Of course, all the meals prepared are calculated to maintain a negative caloric balance for the participants' size, so weight loss is a physiologic certainty — IF the program is followed.

Buried deep in the Jenny Craig web site is a FAQ section about exercise.

> Jenny Craig's exercise component was developed in consultation with the world-renowned Cooper Institute and encourages clients to gradually increase activity through a combination of natural, planned and playful physical activities..Your Jenny Craig consultant will work with you to develop a personalized, staged approach that starts where you are right now and builds from there...
>
> Research has shown that an active lifestyle is a critical factor in successful weight loss. While it's true that physical activity supports consistent weight loss, its role is even more critical in long-term weight loss.

Jenny Craig admits that an active lifestyle (exercise) is a "critical" factor in successful weight loss. According to the

UCLA and NIH review studies, exercise is likely the ONLY factor — no matter what the diet.

The FAQ goes on:

> In research conducted by the National Weight Control Registry of 4500 individuals who have lost at least 30 pounds and kept it off for one year, it was found that such individuals, on average, are physically active for 60 minutes a day.

The National Weight Control Registry (NWCR) pops up regularly as a reference in diet-based studies. The name, however, is misleading. The NWCR is not associated with the national government. It is a totally voluntary online database with no independent verification of the self-reported data from the "allegedly" formerly-obese.

That said, JC correctly relates the NWCR data that those individuals who have successfully kept off 30 pounds or more long term report exercising for 60 minutes a day on average.

But it is very likely that anyone who exercises for 60 minutes a day will lose weight — with or without Jenny Craig.

Take Home Points

Diet-only weight loss programs are long-term failures for the vast majority of participants, and exercise-based weight loss programs are effective only as long as the individual exercises.

These two approaches both share a common flaw — neither deals adequately with the psychological aspect of hunger or challenges cultural myths about meal consumption.

Chapter 5 The Case for Breakfast Cereal

"You can't skip lunch! Why, it's the most important meal of the day!"

No one ever says that, do they?

The reason is that while most everyone eats a meal at midday, over 20% of American adults routinely skip breakfast.

You can bet that the folks who make breakfast food don't like that one bit. To counter the alarming trend, a myth was created and perpetuated, and breakfast became the most important meal of the day.

The ready-to-eat cereal (RTEC) business is dominated by Kellogg's and General Mills. Their profit margin on cereal is substantial.

Sales for breakfast cereal alone in 2011 totaled 11 billion dollars, and advertising by these companies is likely a double digit percentage of that number. The breakfast cereal ads are subtly or not-so-subtly embedded in nearly every aspect of our culture. The message is appealing and outwardly logical. We must eat a nutritious breakfast!

But why breakfast?

"Early to bed and early to rise makes a man healthy, wealthy, and wise" is an accepted truism, but nowhere does Benjamin Franklin mention the eating of breakfast. You could make just as good a case that everyone should eat a nutritious lunch, or a nutritious dinner. In fact, any meal that is the most nutritious of the day can justifiably be called the most important.

But is the eating breakfast in and of itself necessary for optimal functioning? As we have seen from earlier chapters, the physiologic answer is no—though the cereal companies have sponsored numerous studies trying to prove otherwise. To get around the lack of scientific evidence, these companies resort to linking solid American values—success through hard work, productivity, and a healthy life-style—to the eating of breakfast in their advertisements.

But is this a legitimate connection?

Children, Adolescents, and Breakfast

A caveat: for children and adolescents who are in the growing phase, no one will argue that breakfast should not be eaten. The Essene Diet is not intended to apply to overweight children and adolescents.

However, that said, with the alarming rise in childhood obesity, one can't help but wonder. In life on the farm just two or three generations ago, how many hundreds of calories would an average farm kid burn off doing chores in the morning before eating breakfast? Then, ADHD and autism were unknown maladies. Were these conditions under-diagnosed then, or are the dietary and behavior patterns of today's children a contributing factor to their recent emergence?

Adults and Breakfast

For healthy adults over 20 there are no studies that show that the ritual of an early morning meal is essential or even needed. But breakfast ads routinely show adults happily crunching away on breakfast cereal — implying that they would not be where they are today without it. Adult cultural icons are pictured eating breakfast with relish which encourages impressionable children to do the same. How can health conscious adults not be affected as well, perhaps making a "nutritious" breakfast a part of their own lives even if they have no children to set examples for?

Studies and Studies

With so many American adults routinely skipping breakfast for so many years, negative health consequences resulting from it surely should be apparent by now, but that is not the case.

Undeniably, however, a negative health trend is that America is getting fatter, with 60% of Americans in the overweight category (25-30 BMI) and 20% in the obese category (>30 BMI).

A major focus of many researchers, some with breakfast food industry connections, is to link breakfast-skipping with the development of obesity. But logically, how can skipping breakfast make people fatter? Missing a meal should make people slimmer.

The usual tortured hypothesis is that missing breakfast upsets some internal equilibrium which then turns people into eating machines for the rest of the day. Over time, obesity results. However, this theory has never even come close to being proven — but not for lack of trying.

To investigate eating patterns and obesity, hundreds of nutritional studies have been done involving all aspects of food intake in both children and adults. Most are epidemiologic in nature, where vast data bases are analyzed looking for associations. Very few of these studies find scientifically significant connections of any sort, much less proving that missing breakfast causes obesity. You can recognize these specious studies by the headlines the study might generate. Waffle words such as "linked", "suggested", "may", and "associated" are routinely seen.

Fortunately, it is unnecessary to undertake an exhaustive review of the literature on the subject. The cereal companies have done that for us. On their websites, studies are referenced that support their contention that eating breakfast is good for adults. Presumably, these studies are the best of the lot.

But before we look at them, let us first spend a few chapters learning about human physiology, metabolics, and biochemistry.

Chapter 6 Biochemistry Essentials

An understanding of biochemistry is needed to appreciate how the human body works. While the subject might appear daunting, only about 10 elements, or atoms, are dealt with — though these elements are arranged in complex structures and involved in dynamic systems. Just five of these elements are of immediate concern to us: hydrogen, oxygen, carbon, nitrogen, and phosphorus. These atoms make up most of the molecules that were introduced in the second chapter — glucose, amino acids, fats, and ATP.

The world of atoms and molecules is truly alien to our everyday experience. The diameter of a single hydrogen atom is one hundred millionth of a centimeter — extraordinarily small. Even more amazing, if that single hydrogen atom were to travel in a straight line unimpeded, its speed would be 3,000 miles an hour. All atoms possess energies on a similar scale.

Biochemical Energy

Biochemical energy is nuclear in origin and comes from the sun. Only a tiny fraction of the sun's radiation is captured in plant chemical bonds — this through the process of photosynthesis. Photosynthesis first developed 3.4 billion years ago. The energy from oil comes from its carbon-hydrogen (C-H) bonds which themselves were originally created by photosynthetic reactions in growing plants tens of millions of years ago. While the plants died, became buried, and were transformed physically into oil, their energy-laden C-H bonds remained intact.

Humans and animals cannot use the energy from the sun directly, but they do eat plants and so pirate the plant's bond energy. When animals eat other animals or humans eat animals, bond energy is similarly transferred.

The Basics of Atoms and Bonding

Atoms are the building blocks of life and matter. Atoms have a positively charged nucleus made up of neutrons and protons. The neutron and the proton have an equal mass but the proton carries a positive charge where the neutron is neutral. Surrounding the positively charged nucleus are "shells" of electrons. An electron is a thousand times smaller than a proton, but carries an equal though negative electrical charge. In an atom, the number of protons and electrons are usually the same, giving the atom an over-all neutral charge.

Hydrogen has only one proton in its nucleus and one electron in its single shell. To give an idea of scale, the hydrogen atom is 100,000 times larger than the size of its single proton core, and 100 million times larger than its single electron. In fact, atoms are composed of mostly empty space — demonstrating how relatively powerful the electric charges in protons and electrons are.

An atom can have several layers of shells filled with electrons. The number of available electrons in the atom's outermost shell determines the number of bonds the atom can form. The most important type of bond in biochemistry, for our purposes, is the covalent bond. This is where electrons are shared between two atoms. Essentially, there is a partial merger between the outermost shells of the atoms. It is in these bonds where energy is stored. When a bond is broken, the energy is released as heat or transferred into another bond through a coupled biochemical reaction.

Water

Water is the basis of life. Almost all biochemical reactions take place in a sea of water molecules, and water is assumed to be a co-factor in every biochemical reaction. Life evolved from the ocean, so this makes sense.

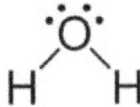

Above is a single water molecule. To gain an appreciation of scale, a single cubic centimeter of water contains 30 billion trillion individual water molecules.

We see here and on page 41 that two hydrogen atoms ("H") are bonded to a central oxygen atom ("O") by covalent single bonds. Each bond line represents two electrons — one contributed by the hydrogen atom (it has only one) and one from the oxygen atom.

The two pairs of dots on the upper pole of the oxygen atom represent the two "lone" pairs of electrons in oxygen's outer shell. These electrons are happy just to resonate together without getting involved in bonding. Electrons can be compared to spinning tops. Two with opposite spins will attract each other and resonate, and so will not bond with the electrons of other atoms.

The Oxygen Atom

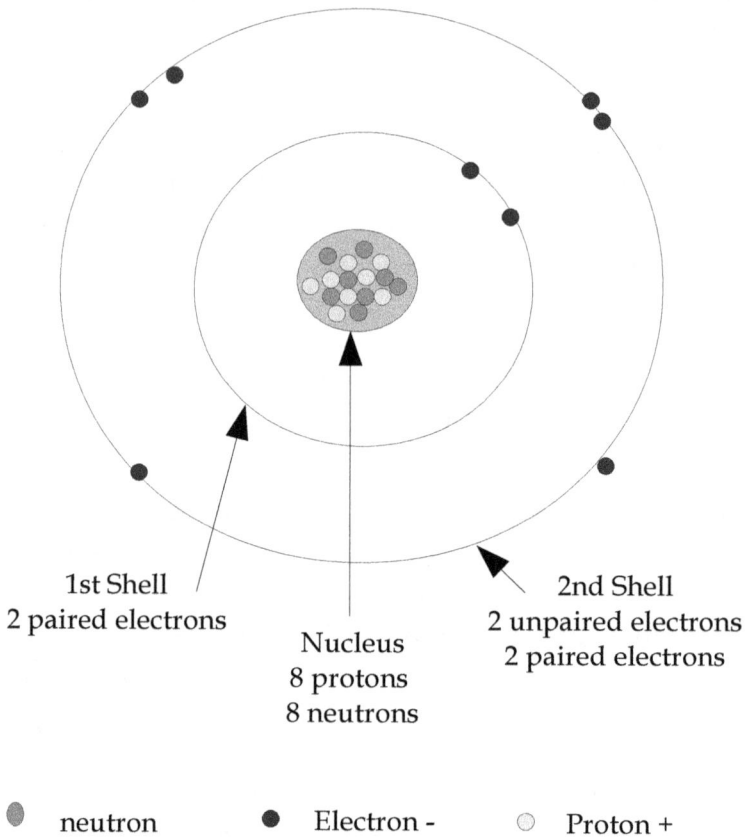

1st Shell
2 paired electrons

Nucleus
8 protons
8 neutrons

2nd Shell
2 unpaired electrons
2 paired electrons

● neutron   ● Electron -   ○ Proton +

Oxygen has an atomic number of 8 which means that the
neutral oxygen atom has 8 neutrons and 8 protons in its
nucleus, and 8 total electrons-2 in the first shell and 6 in the
second shell. In the outer shell, 4 of these electrons are
spin-paired. Paired electrons are not available for bonding.

The Water Molecule
H_2O

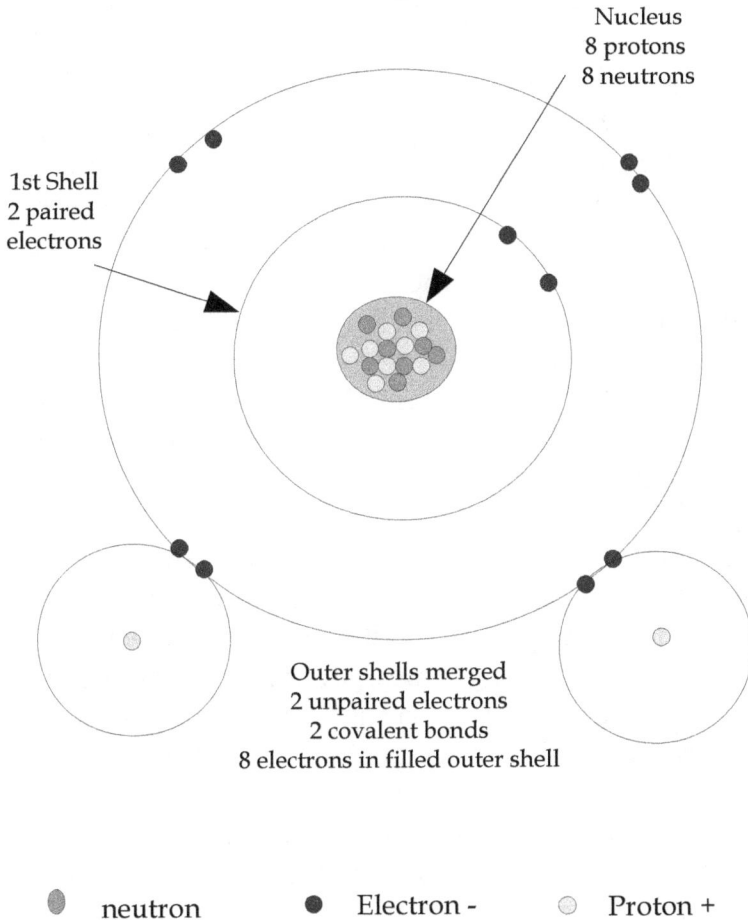

Nucleus
8 protons
8 neutrons

1st Shell
2 paired
electrons

Outer shells merged
2 unpaired electrons
2 covalent bonds
8 electrons in filled outer shell

neutron   Electron -   Proton +

Hydrogen has an atomic number of 1 which means it has 1 proton in its nucleus and 1 electron in a single shell. The water molecule H_2O has an atomic weight of 18. The hydrogen nuclei stay to one side of the molecule, with the two lone pairs of electrons on the other side. This produces an asymmetric charge and a "polar" molecule.

The oxygen atom has six electrons in its outer shell, but only two are unpaired and available for bonding. In comparison, nitrogen (N) has three unpaired electrons and a single resonating electron pair, phosphorous (P) has five unpaired electrons, and carbon (C) has four.

The water molecule illustrates the important concept of polarity. The two lone pairs of electrons on the upper pole of our molecule lend an overall negative charge to it. On the opposite pole, the electrons involved in the O-H bonds tend to spend most of their time between the nucleus of the hydrogen and oxygen atoms. This means that the positive hydrogen nucleus is more "exposed" and not shielded by the negatively charged electron. This lends a positive charge to that aspect of the molecule, giving water its strong electrical asymmetry, or "polarity."

Larger molecules are similar, having unique three-dimensional "fold-over" conformations due to their electrical charges. These same characteristics determine their reactive properties with other molecules — cell membrane receptors, enzymes, or reaction substrate. A molecule can easily be thousands of times larger than our water molecule with a corresponding increase in the complexity of its conformation and charge distribution.

The polarity factor is how liquid water can dissolve solid masses of other molecules. The small polar water molecules "attack" the pack molecules and orient themselves around each of them according to the target molecules' charge pattern — with unlike charges attracting and like charges repelling. If the molecules in the solid are polar enough, they can separate out from the pack by the action of intervening water molecules, and so the pack "dissolves."

Carbohydrates and amino acids are sufficiently polar to dissolve in aqueous solutions while lipids are not. In fact, it is this property of insolubility in water that defines a lipid.

For this reason, fats need a different mode of digestion by the human gastrointestinal system, as will be outlined. Also, being resistant to the dissolving action of water, lipids are ideally suited to make up the cell membrane.

Carbon

Life is also carbon-based and for a good reason. Unlike other atoms, carbon is uniquely capable of forming long chains by making stable bonds with itself. If complex life is found on other planets, it will likely be based on carbon. To give an idea of scale, a cubic centimeter of pure carbon contains 100 billion trillion individual atoms.

The carbon atom has four electrons in its outer shell, and, unlike oxygen, all of these electrons are available for bonding — there is no need to worry about lone pairs.

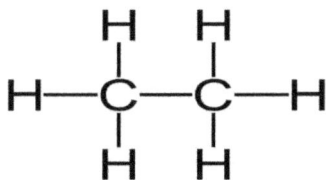

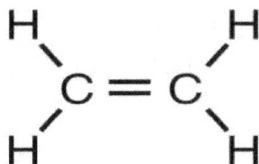

Ethane (left) results when two carbon atoms are joined by a single bond, and the three remaining carbon outer shell electrons bond to hydrogen. Double bonds are possible, as in ethylene (right) where the two carbons share four electrons between them. The remaining electrons are bonded to hydrogen.

Triple bonds (acetylene) are also possible but are rarely seen in biochemistry. The triple bond holds more energy than the double bond, which holds more energy than the single bond.

The Carbon Atom

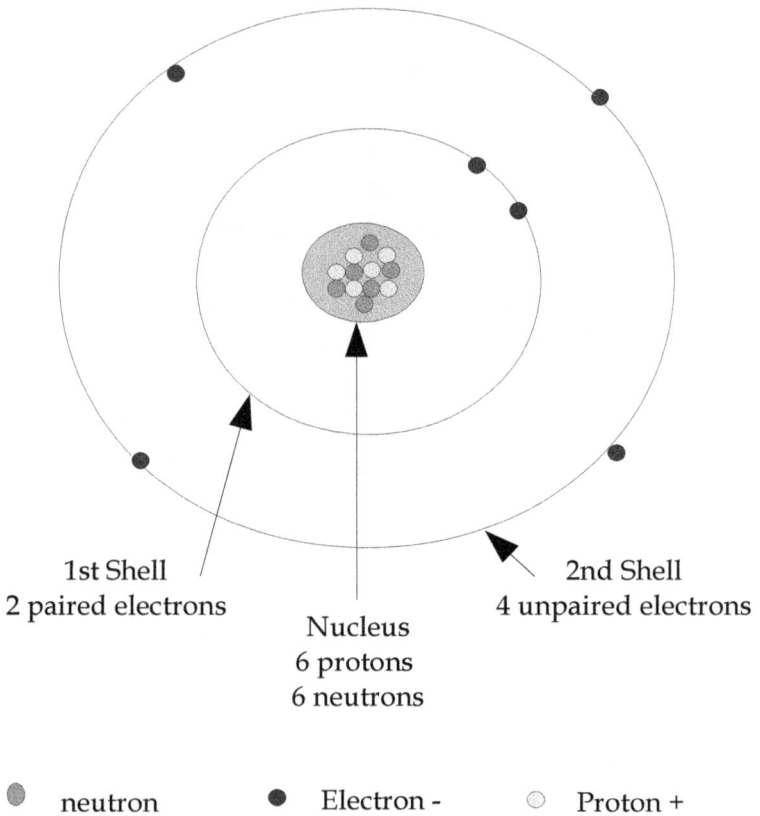

1st Shell
2 paired electrons

Nucleus
6 protons
6 neutrons

2nd Shell
4 unpaired electrons

⬤ neutron   ⬤ Electron -   ○ Proton +

Carbon has an atomic number of 6 which means that the neutral carbon atom has 6 neutrons and 6 protons in its nucleus, and 6 electrons in two shells surrounding the nucleus. In its outermost shell carbon has four unpaired electrons available for bonding.

Digested carbohydrates are processed in the liver and released into the serum as 95% glucose.

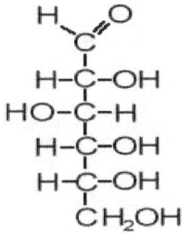

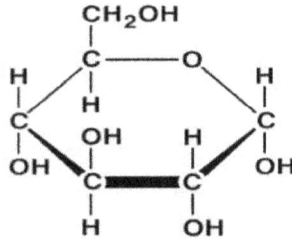

In the serum, the 6-carbon glucose is in cyclic form.

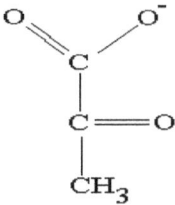

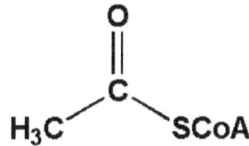

Glucose can be broken down into two molecules of pyruvate (left) made of three carbon atoms each. Pyruvate can be broken down to acetyl-CoA (right) which is the "entry" molecule for all oxidative energy production.

Excess glucose is packaged into a storage polymer called glycogen (next page). Glycogen is a highly branched molecule and forms granules in the cell.

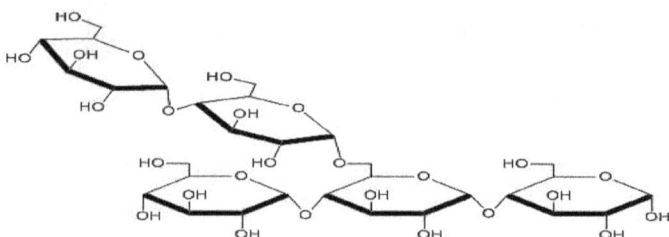

Below is adenosine tri-phosphate, or ATP. This is the energy currency of the cell and the true fuel of the body. The energy derived from the breaking of the C-H bonds in organic molecules is transferred into two P-O bonds of the ATP molecule.

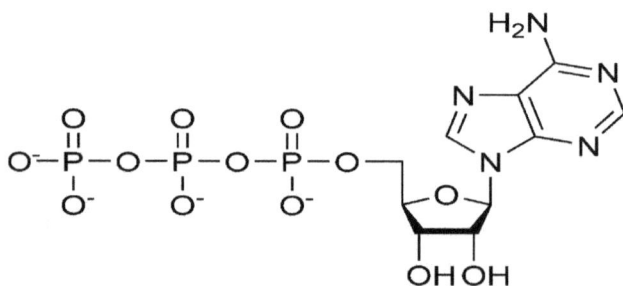

Lipids (fats)

Lipids are defined by their being insoluble in water. Triglycerides, cholesterol, and phospholipids are all fats.

On the next page is a molecule of palmitic oil, a neutral triglyceride (TG). Three 16-carbon fatty acid (FA) chains are joined by ester linkages (C-O-C) to a 3-carbon glycerol (GLY) base on the left. TGs make up most fat tissue. The number of C-H bonds makes it easy to see why fats have over twice the energy per unit mass as does carbohydrates.

```
              O    H  H  H  H  H  H  H  H  H  H  H  H  H  H  H  H
   H           \\   |  |  |  |  |  |  |  |  |  |  |  |  |  |  |  |
   |            C -C -C -C -C -C -C -C -C -C -C -C -C -C -C -C -H
 H-C-O        /    |  |  |  |  |  |  |  |  |  |  |  |  |  |  |  |
   |                H  H  H  H  H  H  H  H  H  H  H  H  H  H  H  H
   |          O    H  H  H  H  H  H  H  H  H  H  H  H  H  H  H  H
   |           \\   |  |  |  |  |  |  |  |  |  |  |  |  |  |  |  |
 H-C-O          C -C -C -C -C -C -C -C -C -C -C -C -C -C -C -C -H
   |          /    |  |  |  |  |  |  |  |  |  |  |  |  |  |  |  |
   |                H  H  H  H  H  H  H  H  H  H  H  H  H  H  H  H
   |          O    H  H  H  H  H  H  H  H  H  H  H  H  H  H  H  H
   |           \\   |  |  |  |  |  |  |  |  |  |  |  |  |  |  |  |
 H-C-O          C -C -C -C -C -C -C -C -C -C -C -C -C -C -C -C -H
   |          /    |  |  |  |  |  |  |  |  |  |  |  |  |  |  |  |
   H                H  H  H  H  H  H  H  H  H  H  H  H  H  H  H  H
```

The breaking apart of the neutral triglyceride into "free" fatty acids (FFA) and glycerol (GLY) involves the addition of a water molecule to break each ester linkage. Glycerol ends up with three alcohol groups (OH), and each of the three FFAs has a carboxylic acid group (COOH) on one end. To reconstruct the triglyceride, the same atoms have to be removed from the GLY and FFAs, producing three molecules of water as well as the TG.

A fatty acid chain is "saturated" if all the carbon-carbon bonds are single and "unsaturated" if one or more of the C-C bonds are double. A C=C double bond changes the conformation of the molecule and hence its properties. An unsaturated fatty acid is below.

```
    O    H  H  H  H  H  H    H  H  H
     \\  |  |  |  |  |  |     |  |  |
      C -C -C -C -C -C -C =C -C -C
     /   |  |  |  |  |          \  C-H
    O    H  H  H  H  H          / |
    |                          H  H
    H
```

Note the double bond and the resulting change in the carbon skeleton angle. In adipose tissue which is composed of billions of fat cells, when the temperature drops the percentage of unsaturated fatty chains naturally increases as a result. This serves to decrease the density of the fats and lower the melting point, so the fats remain in liquid form instead of solidifying.

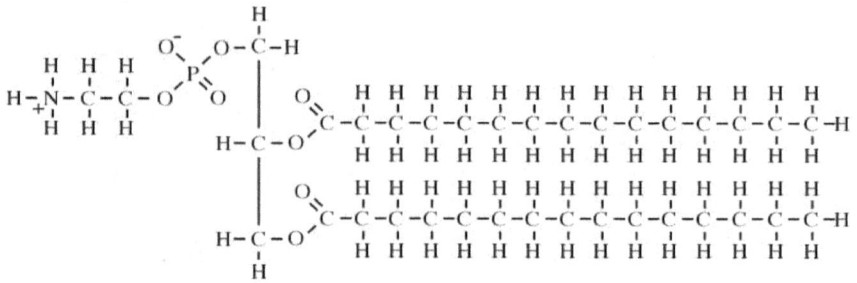

Above is lecithin, which is an example of a phospholipid. The central GLY molecule has only two FA chains attached by ester linkages. The third GLY carbon is bonded to a phosphate group, which itself is bonded to a another chemical group which defines the type of phospholipid that it is. This type of bi-polar molecule is a key part of structural elements in all cell membranes.

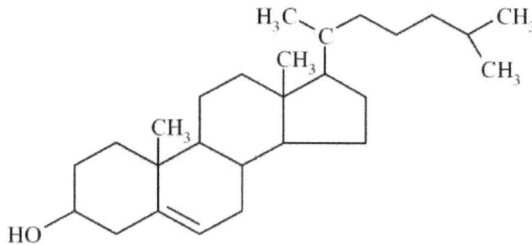

Cholesterol, above, is made in the liver from individual molecules of 2-carbon acetyl-CoA. Cholesterol serves as an important constituent of cell membranes and bile acids — which are made in the liver and stored in the gall bladder. Cholesterol is the base for all of the steroid hormones.

Amino Acids

Proteins are broken down in the gastrointestinal tract to amino acids and absorbed. Like carbohydrates, they are polar molecules and are soluble in water. In an amino acid, different groups are bonded to a "central" carbon atom.

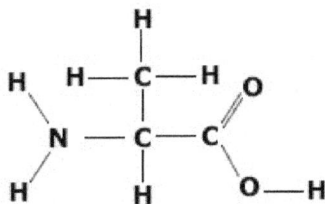

Alanine, above, is the simplest amino acid. An amino group (NH2) and a carboxylic acid group (COOH) are bonded to a central carbon atom along with a single hydrogen atom. Each amino acid also has an "R" group attached to the central carbon which can vary and defines the type of amino acid that it is. In alanine, the R group is CH3, or methane. Amino acids can be linked in chains through "peptide" bonds between their amino and carboxylic acid groups and so form proteins.

The Cell

The human body is made of an astounding total of 100 trillion cells that work together in functional coordination. All of these cells originated from a single "mother" cell that underwent many generations of division and differentiation. If it were possible to line up end-to-end all the cells in a human being, the resulting chain would circle the earth three times!

A cell with a nucleus and mitochondria developed about 2 billion years ago. To put that into perspective, 600 million years ago simple animals evolved. Mammals showed up about 200 million years ago. The first primitive man-like creature came on the scene 2.5 million years ago, with the anatomically "modern" humanoid appearing in the fossil

The Cell Made Very Simple

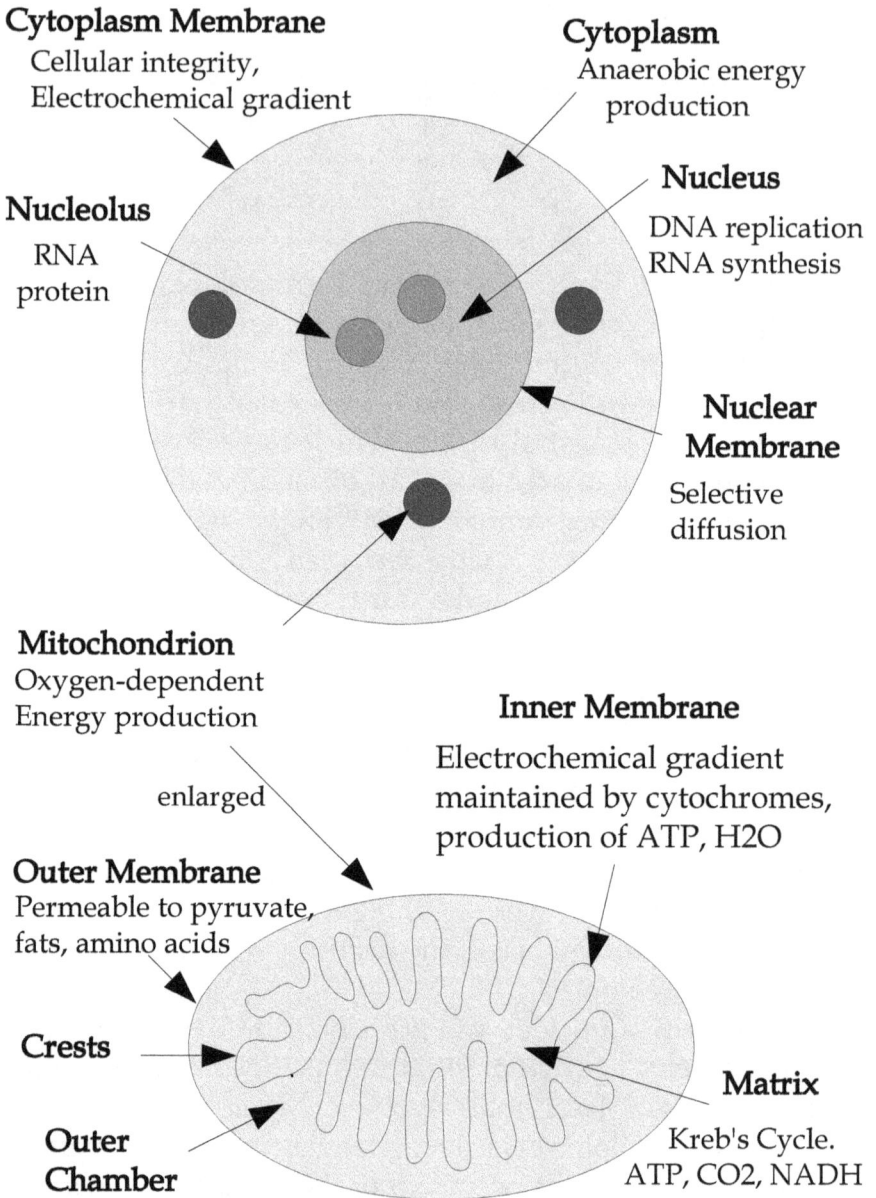

Cytoplasm Membrane
Cellular integrity,
Electrochemical gradient

Cytoplasm
Anaerobic energy
production

Nucleolus
RNA
protein

Nucleus
DNA replication
RNA synthesis

**Nuclear
Membrane**
Selective
diffusion

Mitochondrion
Oxygen-dependent
Energy production

Inner Membrane
Electrochemical gradient
maintained by cytochromes,
production of ATP, H_2O

enlarged

Outer Membrane
Permeable to pyruvate,
fats, amino acids

Crests

**Outer
Chamber**

Matrix
Kreb's Cycle.
ATP, CO_2, NADH

record 200,000 years ago. Evidence for Cro-Magnon man — us! — goes back 20,000 years.

All human cells function basically the same, and all have individual specialized roles to play. The cell is surrounded by a lipid bi-layer membrane that is selectively permeable to various substances. This allows for separate fluid compartments to be maintained. Embedded in these membranes, along with protein enzymes and receptor molecules, are sodium-potassium "pumps" that create and maintain an electrochemical gradient between the outside "interstitial" fluid and the cell's interior or "cytoplasm."

Almost two-thirds of the energy used by the body at rest is consumed by these membrane pumps. The cell, in fact, can be compared to a very small battery. With trillions of cells, the potential energy adds up quickly. This "battery" power is important in the transmission of impulses in nerve cells, the contraction of muscle cells, glandular secretions, and other functions.

Most cells have a centrally-located nucleus where the DNA is located and where the RNA templates for protein synthesis are made. The nucleus is set apart from the cytoplasm by its own lipid bilayer membrane.

In the cytoplasm, proteins are synthesized for the cell's own use or for export. Also, energy can be produced anaerobically through glycolysis. Not pictured in the simple cell diagram are most of the cell's internal machinery such as the Golgi apparatus, endoplasmic reticulum, ribosomes, peroxisomes, lysosomes, etc.

Adipose tissue is made of modified fibroblast cells. These cells contain enzymes that allow them to obtain, process, and store triglycerides in their cytoplasm. An "empty" fat cell can potentially swell to 20 times its original size by storing liquid triglycerides — a "fat" cell, indeed!

The Mitochondrion

An important membrane-enclosed organelle in the cell cytoplasm is the mitochondrion. It is in the mitochondrion where most of the ATP is produced, and the only place in the cell where ATP can be produced with the use of oxygen. Without the mitochondrion, the cells ability to make ATP would be cut by at least 90%. In fact, the "modern" cell would not be able to exist.

There can be hundreds and even thousands of mitochondria organelles in the cytoplasm of any one cell. Across the inner membrane of the mitochondrion an electrochemical gradient is maintained by hydrogen ion "pumps." This electrical potential powers the eventual synthesis of ATP. The mitochondrion, like the larger cell itself, can be thought of as a small battery.

Amazingly, the mitochondria have their own DNA/RNA systems and can self-replicate under certain conditions. In muscle cells, regular exercise can cause a 60% or more increase in the number of energy-producing mitochondria.

Because of the ability to self-replicate, it has been postulated that mitochondria started out as a separate cells billions of years ago. Through a chance mutation, a symbiotic relationship formed between one mitochondrion and an "acceptor" nucleated cell with their genomes combining. The competitive advantage made the mutated cell flourish and dominate.

Take Home Points

Atoms bond together to form molecules. The electrical polarity of molecules determines their shape and properties.

Energy is stored in these bonds. When the bonds are broken, energy is released as heat or transformed into other bonds.

Carbohydrates, fats, and protein are made from simple carbon molecules.

Carbohydrates and protein can dissolve in water while fats do not.

The basic unit of life is the cell. The human body has 100 trillion cells.

Each cell can be thought of as a small battery — the battery power being used to power specific cellular functions.

The mitochondria are small membrane-bound units within each cell that can divide on their own. Mitochondria create 90% of the cell's ATP using oxygen. The mitochondria, too, can be thought of as small batteries.

Most of the bond energy gained by the breakdown of ingested food is used to maintain the electric gradient across the "battery" membranes of both the cells and the mitochondria.

Chapter 7 Digestion

Humans can consume an astonishing variety of substances and thrive. As we learned in chapter 2, all of these foodstuffs can be broken down into three basic "pre-fuels" — carbohydrates, fats, and proteins (amino acids). When needed, these substances can be metabolized aerobically into carbon dioxide and water in the process of making the energy currency of the body, ATP.

Carbohydrates (HT2)

Carbohydrates are composed of starches (rice, potatoes, root vegetables, corn, cereals, breads, etc) and sugars (fruits, vegetables, sugar, pastries, chocolate, soft drinks, etc).

After consumption, carbohydrates are broken down over 1-2 hours in the small intestine to 6-carbon (6-C) molecules called monosaccharides — galactose, fructose, glucose — and released into the hepatic portal vein system. At this point, glucose makes up 80% of the sugars. The liver serves as the "first stop" processor for nutrients and other substances absorbed through the villi of the small intestine. The liver is also a detoxifying agent for noxious substances that might have been ingested. In the liver, all of the galactose and most of the fructose is transformed into glucose. What leaves the liver for the circulation proper is 95% glucose.

Carbohydrate Digestion

Starches- potatoes, grains
Sucrose-cane or beet sugar
Lactose-milk
Cellulose-indigestible

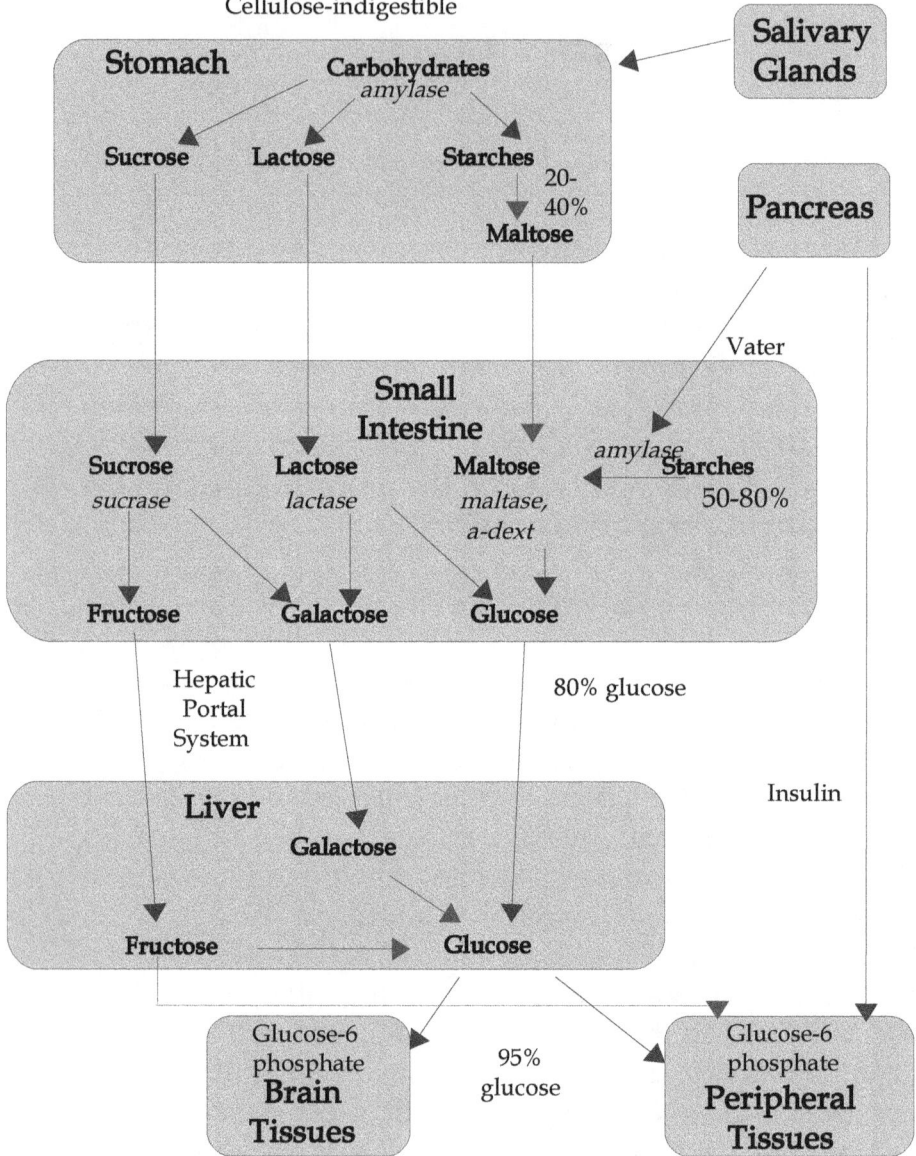

Salivary Glands

Stomach

Carbohydrates
amylase

Sucrose   Lactose   Starches
20-
40%
Maltose

Pancreas

Vater

Small Intestine

Sucrose   Lactose   Maltose   *amylase* Starches
sucrase   *lactase*   *maltase,*   50-80%
                        a-dext

Fructose   Galactose   Glucose

Hepatic
Portal
System

80% glucose

Insulin

Liver

Galactose

Fructose ———→ Glucose

Glucose-6
phosphate
**Brain
Tissues**

95%
glucose

Glucose-6
phosphate
**Peripheral
Tissues**

Cellulose is an indigestible carbohydrate that is passed through the digestive tract unprocessed. Many diet foods use cellulose as a bulking agent in order to give the stomach the sensation of satiety without adding to the net caloric load.

Some experts blame the increase in childhood obesity on the cumulative effect of fructose exposure to the liver. Over the past 20 years, high-fructose corn syrup has become the sweetener of choice in most soft drinks. But a causative link is unlikely to established. The previous sweetener was sucrose which itself was composed of 50% fructose. This compares to 75% fructose in "high" fructose corn syrup — not much difference. Plus, phosphorylated fructose is a ubiquitous intermediary in cellular glycolysis and in the pentose phosphate pathway, both of which produce ATP.

Glucose

The level of serum glucose is strictly regulated. Receptors in the alpha and beta cells of the pancreas and, less importantly, the neurons of the feeding and satiety centers in the brain's hypothalamus are exquisitely sensitive to blood glucose levels. If the level varies even minutely from the normal baseline level of 70-90 mg/dl (milligrams per deciliter of serum), hormones are released immediately to correct it.

Glucose is the preferred fuel for all of the cells, but too high of a concentration of free glucose can cause trans-membrane fluid-shift abnormalities as well as the glycosylation of other molecules. Brain cells are freely permeable to glucose and so are especially at risk.

When there is an oversupply of glucose, liver and muscle cells have the capability to link up glucose molecules in a compact polymer form called glycogen — as we saw in the previous chapter. The average glycogen molecule is composed of 40,000 glucose molecules connected in branched chain formation. Glycogen then precipitates out in the cell cytoplasm as discrete granules.

Glycogen can make up as much as 8 percent of the liver's total weight, and as much as 3 percent of the body's total muscle mass—a 30-70 absolute ratio. Taken together, the weight of a "full boat" of body glycogen is about 300 milligrams, or less than a pound—but enough to supply the body's baseline glucose needs for 12-24 hours.

When glycogen stores are at maximal levels, the excess glucose is converted into neutral triglycerides (TGs) in the liver. This fat is either stored in the liver or packaged up with other lipids in transport micelles and released into the bloodstream. There, adipose tissue cells will pick up and store the triglycerides—after a further breakdown and resynthesis process.

Lipids (HT3)

Saturated fats are largely of animal origin and are found in significant amounts in food such as beef, butter, cheese, eggs, milk, pork, and palm oil.

Unsaturated fats are of mostly plant origin and include food like avocados, olives, corn oil, soy oil, and margarine. Fish also contains a significant amount of unsaturated fats. The carbon backbone in these fats has a variable number of C=C double bonds.

Lipids are made up of neutral triglycerides (TGs), cholesterol (CHOL), and phosholipids (PLs). A neutral TG molecule is made of three molecules of free fatty acids (FFAs) joined to a glycerol (GLY) base. In the digestion process, the insoluble fats are broken down into small clumps within the chyme of the stomach and then passed into the small intestine. The fats trigger the release of the small intestine hormone cholecystokinin which signals the gall bladder to release bile acids and lethicin. These substances further emulsify the fats while enzymes (lipases) break down the TGs into FFAs and GLY. In the epithelial cells of the small intestine, the TGs are reformed. Most of these TGs, along with CHOL and Pls, are packaged into large transport micelles called chylomicrons and enter the intestinal lymph.

Lymphatic channels exist throughout the body and are designed to carry away debris, proteins, and other substances too large to enter the venous circulation through the cell membrane. The chylomicrons travel in the lymphatic channels from the small intestine and empty into the venous system via the thoracic duct. In the capillaries of the circulation, the chylomicrons interact with the surfaces of cells of the peripheral and adipose tissues and gradually lose their TGs. The chylomicron remnants, now mostly CHOL and PLs, are taken up by the liver and broken down.

In the post-absorptive phase, the liver exports lipids to the serum in the form of small micelles. These are much smaller than chylomicrons and are associated with proteins called lipoproteins whose sole function is to help transport lipids in this form. There are four main types of transport micelles, differentiated by their centrifuge characteristics. Very low density lipoproteins (VLDLs) contain high amounts of triglycerides and moderate amounts of cholesterol and phospholipids. Over time in the circulation, the VLDLs lose some of their triglycerides to the adipose and peripheral cells and are now called intermediate-density lipoproteins (IDLs). When most all of the triglycerides are gone, IDLs become low-density lipoproteins (LDLs). In LDL, cholesterol dominates. High-density lipoprotein (HDL) contains more than 50% protein,

Lipid Absorption

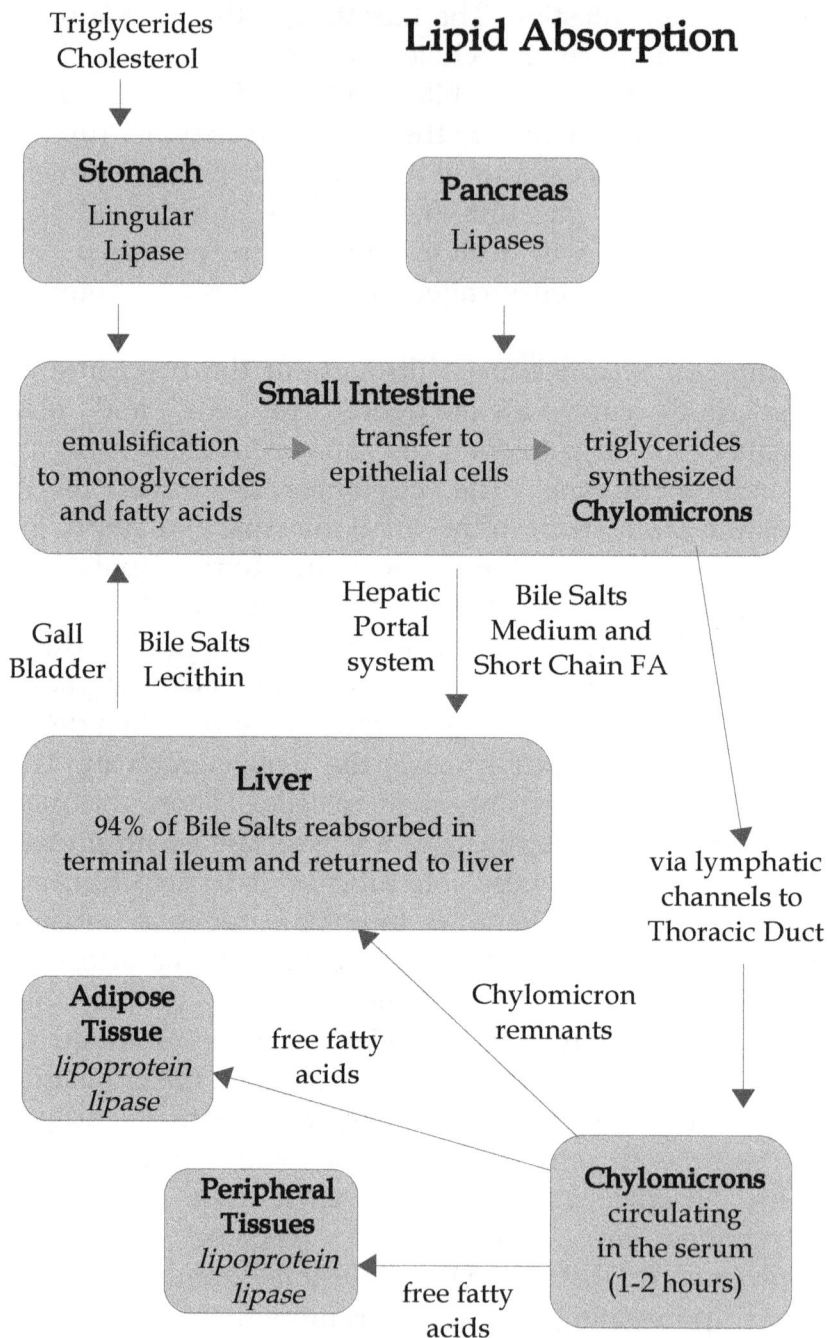

Triglycerides
Cholesterol

Stomach
Lingular
Lipase

Pancreas
Lipases

Small Intestine

emulsification
to monoglycerides
and fatty acids → transfer to
epithelial cells → triglycerides
synthesized
Chylomicrons

Gall
Bladder | Bile Salts
Lecithin

Hepatic
Portal
system

Bile Salts
Medium and
Short Chain FA

Liver
94% of Bile Salts reabsorbed in
terminal ileum and returned to liver

via lymphatic
channels to
Thoracic Duct

**Adipose
Tissue**
*lipoprotein
lipase*

free fatty
acids

Chylomicron
remnants

**Peripheral
Tissues**
*lipoprotein
lipase*

free fatty
acids

Chylomicrons
circulating
in the serum
(1-2 hours)

Lipids in the Post-Absorptive State

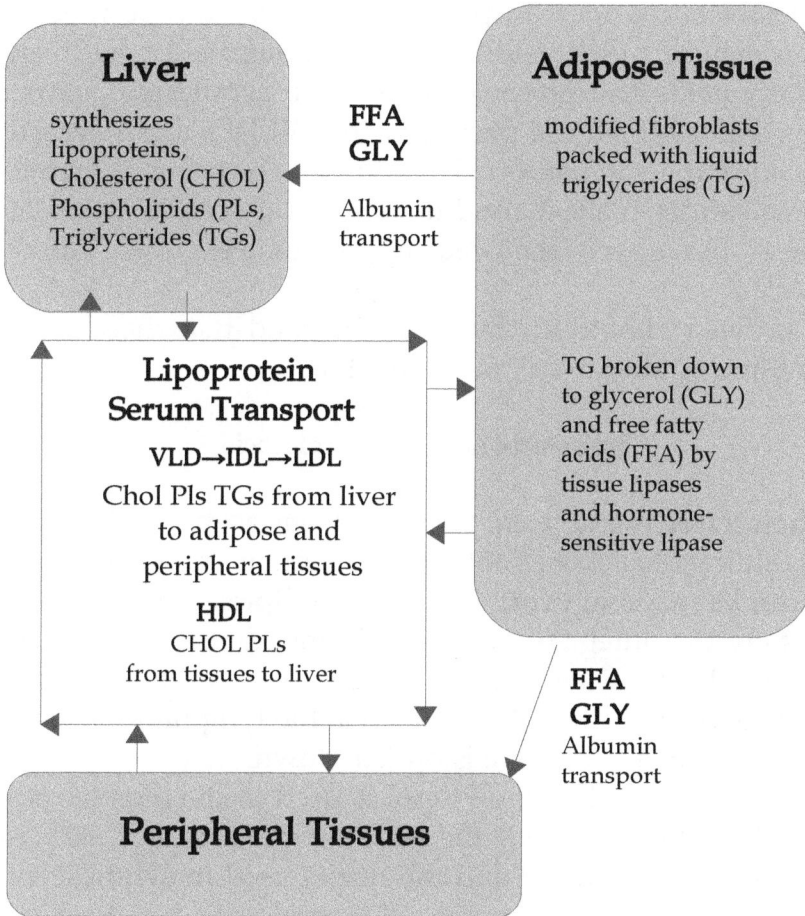

Liver	**Adipose Tissue**
synthesizes lipoproteins, Cholesterol (CHOL) Phospholipids (PLs, Triglycerides (TGs)	modified fibroblasts packed with liquid triglycerides (TG)

FFA
GLY

Albumin
transport

Lipoprotein Serum Transport

VLD→IDL→LDL

Chol Pls TGs from liver
to adipose and
peripheral tissues

HDL
CHOL PLs
from tissues to liver

TG broken down
to glycerol (GLY)
and free fatty
acids (FFA) by
tissue lipases
and hormone-
sensitive lipase

FFA
GLY
Albumin
transport

Peripheral Tissues

and serves to scavenge cholesterol and phospholipids in the body and return them to the liver.

The adipose tissue is constantly releasing FFAs and GLY into the circulation at a rapid rate. Being polar molecules, these substances are transported to the liver and peripheral tissues bound to the plasma protein albumin. In the liver, the fatty acids and glycerol are used to synthesize neutral triglycerides which are packaged into VLDLs and released back into the circulation. Due to this ongoing dynamic process, under normal conditions the triglyceride stores in adipose tissue are renewed approximately every three weeks.

The dieter should always keep in mind that there is no such thing as old fat—all fat is new fat.

Cholesterol and Atherosclerosis

Cholesterol is made in the liver from acetyl-CoA units, the building blocks of all fats. A small amount of CHOL and PLs can be made in every cell, as these lipids are needed to maintain the integrity of the cell membrane. Ingested cholesterol finds its way to the liver as chylomicron remnants from the small intestine via the lymphatic system, as we have seen, and there is broken down.

Most of the body's cholesterol is used in the membranes of its 100 trillion cells. Of the remaining cholesterol, 80% is used to form bile acids, and the rest is used in synthesis of the adrenocortical hormones aldosterone and cortisol, as well as the sex hormones testosterone and estrogen.

Cholesterol plays a significant role in the development of atherosclerotic plaques in arterial blood vessels. Low levels of cholesterol (LDL) in the blood correspond to a lower incidence of heart disease and stroke. A high HDL to LDL ratio is optimal, with the LDL level being kept under 130 mg/dl. However, the pathogenisis of atherosclerosis suggests that cholesterol might only play a supporting role.

The inside of mid-sized and large arteries are protected by a smooth protein coat, and the endothelial cells themselves release NO2 which is also protective. Atherosclerosis begins when damage occurs to the endothelial lining. This can be caused by high blood pressure, infection, or a failure of the endothelium's protective mechanisms. High blood pressure is likely the major culprit, as in the low-pressure venous side of the circulation, atherosclerotic plaques are rarely seen.

Monocytes are primitive white blood cells that are made in the bone marrow and released into the bloodstream. There, they travel about harmlessly looking for any defect in the endothelium. If one is found, the monocytes will adhere to it and try to squeeze through the defect to gain entrance to the inner layers of the vessel wall. If the monocytes are successful, tissue factors in the wall activate the monocytes and turn them into aggressive macrophages — the inflammatory process begins!

The macrophages release messenger molecules, called lymphokines, into the blood. These recruit other cells of inflammation as well as attracting cholesterol-laden LDL micelles. Fibrin is laid down under the endothelium as a result of this process, as well as smooth muscle fibers. The LDLs are consumed by the macrophages which then can swell to five times their size, forming "foam" cells.

Over time the plaques grow with the continued deposition of fibrin, smooth muscle, lipids, and other accumulated debris of inflammation. A plaque can become large enough to narrow the vessel lumen and restrict blood flow. In coronary arteries, this can cause unstable angina if the narrowing is greater than 95%. A plaque can also rupture through the endothelial lining of the vessel causing the arterial blood to coagulate and further narrow the vessel lumen. The clot can break off and become a thrombus which then can totally occlude the vessel further downstream. In coronary arteries, this is called a heart attack. In cerebral arteries, the thrombus causes a stroke.

A primary prevention strategy against atherosclerosis is to prevent the initial damage to the vessel endothelium. This can be done by controlling blood pressure through maintaining a healthy weight, engaging in vigorous physical activity, and not smoking.

Reducing LDL levels is also important. A low-cholesterol diet, however, has only a mild effect on lowering LDL levels. Consumed cholesterol is almost all broken down in the liver. Significantly, this extra load of cholesterol precursors has an over-all depressive effect on the liver's rate of cholesterol synthesis. So the net increase in serum cholesterol after a diet high in cholesterol is not great.

A diet high in saturated fats can increase the serum cholesterol up to 25%. The added acetyl-CoA units in the liver from the breakdown of the saturated triglycerides is thought to be the cause. Conversely, a diet high in unsaturated fats will decrease the cholesterol level moderately through an unknown mechanism.

There are two types of drugs that can lower cholesterol as well. The statins are a group that serve to block a key enzyme in the liver's synthetic pathway of cholesterol and can lower LDL cholesterol 50-75%. Another approach is to bind the bile that is released by the gall bladder by introducing resin agents into the small intestine. The bile salts then cannot be reabsorbed in the terminal ileum and are eliminated through the GI tract. Bile salts are made from cholesterol, so more cholesterol is diverted for that purpose in the liver, with less being released into the serum. Ingesting oat bran has a similar binding effect on bile acids.

Amino Acids (HT4)

The pre-fuel of last resort for the body is protein that has been broken down into amino acids. There are plant and animal proteins. Animal protein includes milk and dairy products as well as meats which usually contain a large amount of fat. Plant protein includes nuts and soy products.

Proteins are soluble in water and so are digested much like carbohydrates. Proteins are broken down in the stomach and small intestine into their constituent amino acids and absorbed directly into the hepatic portal system. The amino acids are taken up by the liver cells from the portal blood, with any residual protein fragments being immediately broken down. Ingested protein that inadvertently reaches the circulation proper can cause a deadly immune response.

Released by the liver into the venous circulation, the amino acids are quickly taken up by the cells and used to form structural elements, hormones, enzymes, etc.

Excess amino acids are transformed in the liver by first removing the nitrogen group and then breaking the carbon skeleton down into either 3-C or 2-C units. Fatty acids or glycerol can be made from them, which are then used to make triglycerides. The TGs are packaged into VLDLs and released into the bloodstream, where they are taken up by the adipose tissue, processed, reformulated, and stored.

Of note is that only 60% of the 20 basic amino acids have the right type of carbon skeleton that can be successfully broken down into these simple carbon units and used for fuel.

Protein Digestion

Proteins are made of a chain of amino acids joined together through peptide bonds. Peptide bonds are broken by the addition of water and formed by the removal of water.

Hydrolysis→ -CONH- + H2O = -COOH + H2N-
Condensation→ -COOH + H2N- = -CONH- + H2O

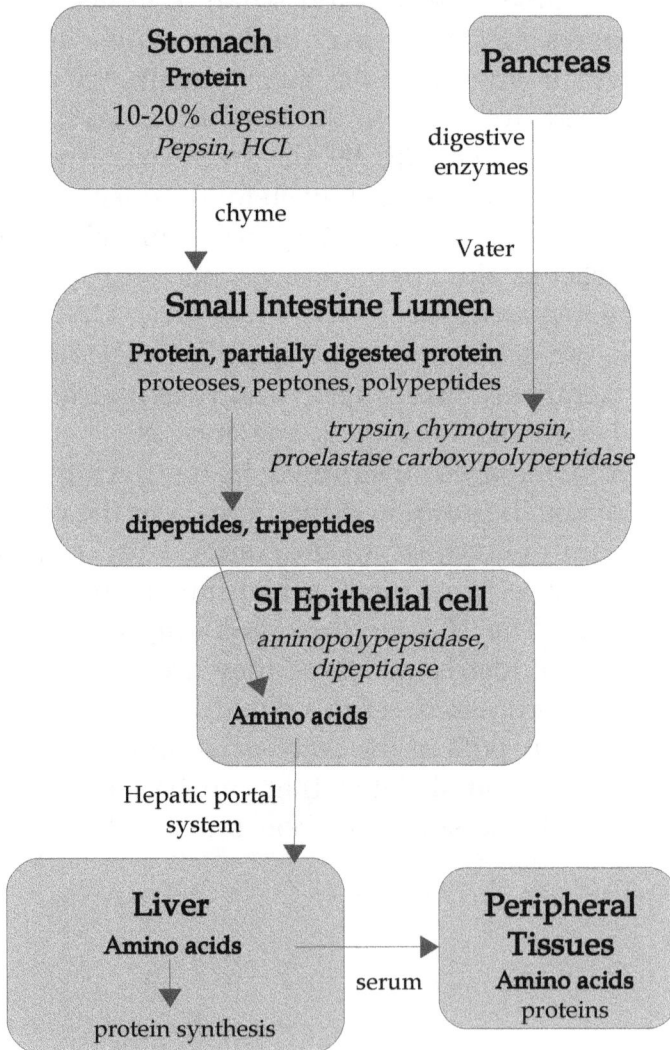

Stomach
Protein
10-20% digestion
Pepsin, HCL

Pancreas

digestive enzymes

chyme

Vater

Small Intestine Lumen

Protein, partially digested protein
proteoses, peptones, polypeptides

trypsin, chymotrypsin,
proelastase carboxypolypeptidase

dipeptides, tripeptides

SI Epithelial cell
aminopolypepsidase,
dipeptidase
Amino acids

Hepatic portal system

Liver
Amino acids
↓
protein synthesis

serum

Peripheral Tissues
Amino acids
proteins

Take Home Points

Virtually all foodstuffs are broken down into basic 6-, 3-, or 2-carbon units for metabolic or synthetic purposes. The human body is in a dynamic state with most of its elements being continuously broken down and resynthesized — though the rates vary considerably. The fat stores in the average human have a high turnover rate, and are totally replaced every 3-4 weeks.

Carbohydrates and proteins are broken down in the stomach and small intestine to basic elements. Being able to be dissolved in water, they are absorbed directly into the hepatic portal system and are processed in the liver before being release into the general circulation.

Lipids, not being soluble in water, are broken down in small intestine and packaged into fatty "micro-droplets" that enter the general circulation through the lymphatic channels. The fats can then be directly absorbed by the adipose or muscle tissue in the capillaries, or brought to the liver for further processing.

Cholesterol is made in the liver. Virtually all cholesterol consumed is broken down into its constituent 2-carbon units and used for cholesterol synthesis or other purposes.

In atherosclerosis, a defect in the endothelial membrane of the arterial vessel wall must first be present in order for the cholesterol-laden plaque to form. One of the major causes of these lesions is high blood pressure.

Chapter 8 Metabolics

Glucose is the cell's fuel of choice probably because, unlike fats or proteins, energy can be extracted from glucose without the presence of oxygen. And even if oxygen is present in the cell, the energy produced anaerobically can be provided much faster—within seconds. It takes the oxidative processes in the mitochondria a minute or so to reach full ATP production.

Anaerobic Metabolism

The anaerobic production of ATP through the breakdown of glucose is called glycolysis. The result is two molecules of pyruvate and two molecules of ATP per glucose molecule. Under anaerobic conditions, the mitochondrial processes are blocked, and so pyruvate builds up in the cell cytoplasm. There, it is converted into lactic acid and in turn diffuses out of the cell and into the serum.

Glycolysis is a fast power source, but it is not an efficient one. Two molecules of ATP are created per molecule of glucose, but 36 more molecules can be produced in the mitochondrion if oxygen is present.

Anaerobic/Aerobic Metabolism

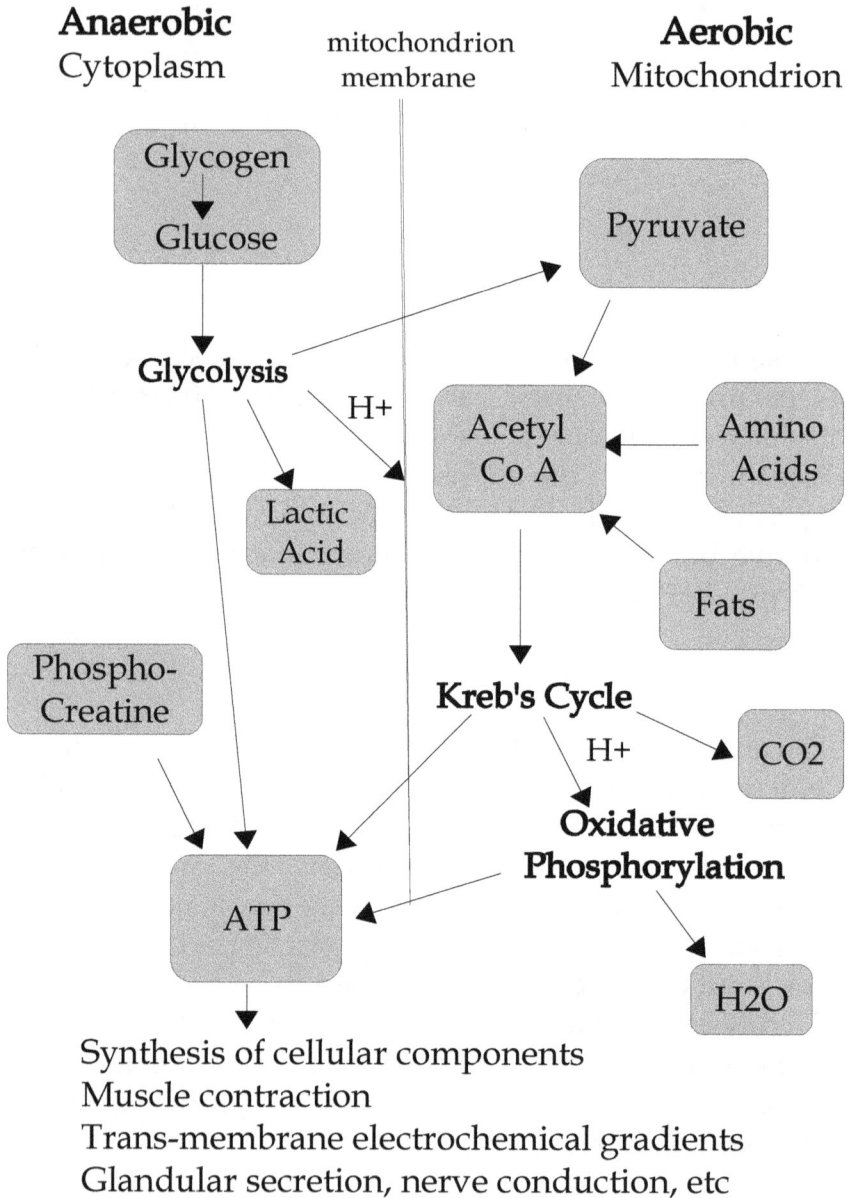

Anaerobic
Cytoplasm

mitochondrion
membrane

Aerobic
Mitochondrion

Glycogen
↓
Glucose

Pyruvate

Glycolysis

H+

Acetyl
Co A

Amino
Acids

Lactic
Acid

Fats

Phospho-
Creatine

Kreb's Cycle

H+

CO_2

**Oxidative
Phosphorylation**

ATP

H_2O

Synthesis of cellular components
Muscle contraction
Trans-membrane electrochemical gradients
Glandular secretion, nerve conduction, etc

When energy is needed quickly — to escape from a charging bear, for instance —, the muscle cell's supply of raw ATP is used up in approximately 2 seconds. After that, the cells' supply of phosphocreatine can be mobilized in a fraction of a second. Taken together, the ATP-phosphocreatine system allows the body to perform at a high level without oxygen for 10 seconds — about the time for a 100 yard dash to safety.

If the bear is still chasing you after 10 seconds, glycogen, the storage form of glucose, is called into play. If the glycogen stores are high, the in-shape human can tap this glucose source and continue in maximal exercise mode for as long as 90 more seconds. Hopefully, 100 seconds will be enough time to escape from the average charging bear.

These three systems together make up the phosphogen system and provide immediate energy while the aerobic system ramps up ATP production. Under these anaerobic conditions, much of the pyruvate produced is converted into lactic acid which diffuses into the blood. Hence, this anaerobic pathway is also termed the glycogen-lactic acid system. The lactic acid in the serum is what causes the fatigue experienced after extreme exertion.

In the unlikely event that the bear is still charging after 100 seconds, ATP should now be being supplied adequately by the mitochondria via the oxidative phosphorylation pathway. If you are in good enough shape, you could gear down to a slow run for an indefinite amount of time to evade the bear — as long as you can resupply yourself with nutrients such as glucose, fats, amino acids, and water.

Oxygen Debt

Assuming that 100 seconds was enough to lose the bear, your lungs are now heaving as you rest. This is because your body is dealing with its "oxygen debt." A depleted phosphogen system requires about 12 liters of oxygen to be reconstituted — the ATP, phosphocreatine, and glycogen have to be regenerated. The respiratory system is stimulated as a result.

The body has only about two liters of oxygen stored at any one time — this being in the lungs, dissolved in the blood, carried by hemoglobin in the blood, or in the muscle tissue. In the average inhalation-exhalation respiratory cycle, the inhaled air has a oxygen concentration of 21%, and the exhaled air has an oxygen concentration of about 16%. So your lungs have their work cut out for them. One liter of oxygen is extracted from the ambient air every 6 respiratory cycles, assuming a three liter volume of air exchange per cycle, so at least 70 heaving breaths are required to supply enough oxygen to reconstitute the phosphogen system. If the volume of air exchange is lower per cycle (normal at rest volume is 500 ml or .5 liters) the number of cycles needed would be correspondingly higher.

In the recharge process, all the lactic acid has to be regenerated into glucose and then to glycogen which consumes ATP. Likewise, the phosphocreatine system has to be replenished requiring ATP production as well. This can take as much as an hour of time.

Fat Metabolism

In the synthesis of ATP in the body's 100 trillion cells, oxygen is consumed, and carbon dioxide and water are released. The oxidative process takes place in the mitochondria of the cell. Both glucose and fats can be broken down to supply the mitochondria with the 2-carbon "entry" molecules it needs to fuel the Kreb's cycle. The specific energy equations, however, are slightly different.

In the breakdown of glucose, 100 molecules of oxygen are used for every 100 molecules of carbon dioxide produced, a 1:1 ratio. With fats, because of the added production of water, only 70 molecules of carbon dioxide are produced for every 100 molecules of oxygen consumed, a .7:1 ratio. This is called the respiratory quotient (RQ) — .7 for fats, and 1.0 for carbohydrates.

Researchers can determine the body's RQ at any given time by carefully monitoring the oxygen and carbon dioxide content of the inhaled and exhaled lung gases in test subjects. They have found that after a meal the RQ is 1.0 and remains so for several hours, indicating that carbohydrates are being metabolized. Fasting, the RQ gradually decreases and after 8-10 hours the RQ is .7. This indicates that the body is now making ATP through the breakdown of fats.

A key element in this switch-over process are low-normal glucose levels due to falling glycogen stores. This is sensed by the hypothalamus in the brain which causes "stress" hormones to be released, which are discussed in the next chapter. These hormones facilitate the body's adaption to fat metabolism as does the drop in insulin levels.

Fats are exclusively metabolized in the mitochondria of the cell. The 3-carbon GLY molecule is converted to pyruvate which is then broken down to a 2-carbon acetyl-CoA molecule which enters the Kreb's cycle. The FA chains have 2-carbon units cleaved off sequentially which are then transformed into acetyl-CoA. This process is called beta oxidation.

The average 70 kg man has 12 kilograms of stored fat in adipose tissue and .3 kilograms of stored glycogen in his liver and muscle tissue. The stored fat can provide 150 times the energy of the stored glycogen.

When the body is fasting and fat is being burned, the glucose levels are still being maintained. The hormone cortisol is important in this process, and it facilitates the breaking down of protein for the purpose of making glucose—a process called gluconeogenisis. The first week in starvation mode, labile proteins (smooth muscle, enzymes) are broken down in order to make glucose. Only after a week of starvation is the more important contractile muscle and brain protein utilized for this purpose.

The rate of free fatty acid (FFA) and glycerol (GLY) release from the adipose tissue is increased by the release of epinephrine from sympathetic stimulation. The free fatty acids and glycerol diffuse easily through the cell membrane of the peripheral tissues, chiefly muscle tissue, and can be used as fuel. The serum FFAs and GLY can also be taken up by the liver and broken down into acetyl-CoA and used for synthesis reactions. If the fasting state lasts for days, the levels of acetyl-CoA in the liver are high enough for it to make 3- and 4-carbon molecules called ketone bodies. These are then released into the serum to be used as fuel by the cells in place of glucose. Interestingly, the brain cells can derive as much as 50-75% of their energy from these ketone bodies under extreme conditions.

In a diabetic crisis, a lack of insulin causes a *de facto* fasting state. Without insulin, glucose cannot enter the cell and so the cell is starving in a sea of glucose! The cell turns to fats for fuel and ultimately ketone bodies are created.

Metabolic Rate

Metabolism refers to all the biochemical reactions that take place in the body. The metabolic rate (MR) measures the rate of heat liberation in the body by these reactions and so is a useful index of energy usage.

Heat is a byproduct of every biochemical reaction. In the aggregate, about 75% of the energy released in these reactions is lost as heat—only 25% is used to make other molecules, maintain electrochemical gradients, or to perform other necessary functions in the body. The metabolic rate is an direct measure of caloric expenditure.

One way to determine the MR is through calorimetry. Test subjects are placed in a special chamber surrounded by water insulation. The increase in water temperature as the person rests reflects directly the body heat loss, and so the rates of biochemical reactions.

There is an indirect way to measure heat loss that is easier to obtain. Oxygen is needed for 95% of the energy-releasing reactions in the body. There is only a slight difference in the amount of heat released between the metabolism of carbohydrates, amino acids, or fats per liter of oxygen consumed. With the same experimental apparatus used to determine the RQ of an individual, the metabolic rate can be calculated with a high degree of precision—using the amount of oxygen extracted by the body over a given time period. On average, one liter of oxygen used accounts for 4.85 Calories of heat lost.

One calorie (small "c") is the amount of heat needed to raise the temperature of one gram of water one degree. As that is a very small amount, for practical reasons kilo-calories are used, which is the amount of energy needed to raise one liter of water (1000 grams, or 1000 milliliters) one degree Celsius. This is called a Calorie (large "C").

At complete rest, the Basal Metabolic Rate (BMR) can be determined which is the minimum level of energy required to maintain life. As energy expenditure is variable among active people, the BMR is useful for comparison purposes.

In the most sedentary of individuals, it accounts for 50-70% of the energy consumed. Skeletal muscle activity is by far the greatest variable in changes in MR. Even at rest, the muscle maintains a tone that requires energy and accounts for 20-30% of the BMR.

A common misconception is that as we age our MR falls as a result of a cellular "wind-down" mechanism. Nothing of this nature, however, has ever been identified. What has been demonstrated is that as people age they lose muscle mass simply due to decreased physical activity. If eating habits are not changed, the muscle is replaced by fat.

Several other factors have an effect on the metabolic rate which we will now discuss.

Thyroxine

Thyroid hormone (thyroxine) can be viewed as a master hormone that responds to external temperature in order to maintain body thermal homeostasis. Thyroxine levels are relatively high in people who live in cold climates, and correspondingly low in those who live in warm climates. Thyroxine works in the nucleus of all cells to set the baseline rate of protein synthesis.

A constant level of thyroxine is maintained by the body, so a drop in levels serves to decrease these rates of reactions and a rise serves to increase them. Practically, this means that essential protein enzyme levels are changed in all cells that can be effected by thyroxine.

Enzymes serve as "templates" upon which two reactants can become properly oriented, enabling a reaction between them to occur. The cell's supply of enzymes is a large factor in the rates of most biochemical reactions. More enzymes — more reactions.

These reactions, however, include both the synthesis and the breakdown of any particular substance, so the net effect is minimal on the substance levels themselves. The amount of heat released in total, however, is variable. Maximal levels of thyroxine can increase the MR 50-100%, while low levels of thyroxine can decrease the MR by 40-60%. These effects are long term, as they take days to develop with any change in thyroxine levels.

Other Influences

Male sex hormones and growth hormone both play a role in muscle growth. The metabolic rate increase can be as much as 15% in those with high testosterone levels, and 20% in those with high growth hormone levels.

Fever is caused by mediators released from white blood cells. These act on the hypothalamic thermo-regulatory centers, with the exact mechanism of heat release unknown. The MR is increased as a result of fever — as much as 120% for every 10 degree Celsius rise in temperature.

Sleep decreases the MR 10-15% through a decrease in muscle tone and a decrease in cerebral activity.

The ingestion of food can increase the MR as reactions take place to digest the food, and as a result of the muscle activity involved in the digestive process itself. The increase in the MR with a fat/carbohydrate meal is 4%. The increase in the MR with a high-protein meal can be up to 30%, with the effect lasting for 3-12 hours.

Malnutrition decreases the MR 20-30% as there is no food to be processed, so no energy is expended in digestive reactions.

Nonshivering Thermogenisis

The factors just discussed cause heat release as a byproduct of their primary function, and not for the sole purpose of producing heat.

There is a process, however, involving certain types of adipose tissue, where heat is the only result—no ATP is produced and this by intention. Initiated through sympathetic stimulation, its purpose is to generate heat in order to protect the body in hypothermic situations.

This speacial type of adipose tissue is called brown fat. The brown fat cells possess many times more energy-producing mitochondria than do normal fat cells. Also, the fat inside the brown cell is stored as many micro-droplets and not just as one large globule as is the case in normal fat cells. Through an unknown mechanism, under sympathetic stimulation the oxidative phosphorylation process in the mitochondria of brown fat becomes uncoupled. Heat is generated, but no ATP is released.

In the infant, brown fat make up about 30% of adipose tissue, and the metabolic rate can increase 100% with maximal sympathetic stimulation. In adults, who have negligible stores of brown fat, this uncoupling process appears to account for about 10% of adipose tissue heat loss under maximal sympathetic stimulation.

The process is being explored as a weigh-loss adjunct, using natural substances (capsaicin, for one) to provide the trigger stimulus. However, with the minimal amount of extra calories burned and the potential negative side effects of the inciting agents, this is not likely to be a long-term weight-control solution.

Exercise

Exercise is by far the most efficient way to burn calories and increase the metabolic rate. For short bursts of strenuous activity the MR can increase over 100 times baseline. In cold conditions, to produce heat the hypothalamus will cause the muscles to shiver — contract purposelessly — in order to harvest the heat produced.

Lying down at complete rest, the average person will burn off 65-70 Calories per hour. If one is standing at rest, this increases to 105 Calories per hour. Walking slowly at 2.6 miles per hour will expend 200 Calories per hour. Running at 5.3 miles per hour burns off 570 Calories per hour, and walking up steps expends 1100 Calories per hour.

Muscles

Skeletal muscles use up a large amount of ATP when they contract. The muscle unit of contraction is called the sarcomere and it is composed of long bundles of actin and myosin protein microfilaments. These are anchored to stationary fibrous bridges at both ends called Z-discs. In a voluntary muscle contraction, the muscle fibers shorten as the actin and myosin microfilaments slide across each other through a rachet-like mechanism — activated by signals from special nerves. The sarcomere unit shortens as a result. These packs of microfilaments can be seen as striations under a microscope hence the name "striated" muscle. Also under the microscope, dense concentrations of mitochondria can be seen close to the filament bundles.

Contractile muscle strength depends upon size. Muscle size is determined by heredity and the level of circulating testosterone. Here, obviously, men have the edge. On average, muscle size is 40% larger in men than in women.

Exercising only minimally increases the levels of circulating testosterone, but through rigorous training muscle size in both sexes can be increased 30-60%. In order for muscles to develop, they must be subject to a load, i.e. they must contract against resistance. This involves the "tearing" of the muscle's microfibrils. In the repair process, the fibrils get bigger. In extreme conditions of exercise, these fibrils can split which further enlarges the muscle.

Researchers have determined that the optimal exercise program for pure muscle strength is six nearly maximal contractions — pick your muscle group — performed three times in a "set" at one session, and this routine repeated three times a week.

As people age and do less work, their strength falls because they lose muscle mass. The initiation of a judicious weight training program can be invaluable for everyone but especially mature adults.

There are two types of muscle fiber — fast-twitch and slow-twitch. Fast-twitch fibers utilize the anaerobic phosphogen system (phosphocreatine-glycogen) twice as efficiently as slow-twitch fibers. Thus, those athletes with a higher percentage of fast-twitch fibers are more proficient in the pure strength events like weightlifting, sprints in track and swimming, and the field events. Those with a higher percentage of slow-twitch fibers are better at the endurance sports such as distance running or swimming.

Slow-twitch fibers are more proficient at utilizing aerobic sources of energy like pyruvate and fatty acids. No amount of training will change this percentage of distribution. The average male has 55% fast-twitch and 45% slow-twitch muscle fibers. The percentage fast-twitch muscle in the average female is probably slightly lower.

Take Home Points

The cells of the body will preferentially utilize glucose for fuel. Glucose can be supplied by glycogen, its storage form.

When the glycogen stores are low, the body will shift over to the burning of fat. For the sedentary or sleeping person, this will occur 8-10 hours after the last meal is consumed.

Oxygen is needed to make most of the ATP the body needs. Without oxygen, ATP can be produced at adequate levels only a few minutes until irreversible cell injury occurs.

The metabolic rate (MR) is a measure of heat and directly indicates the level of metabolic activity in the body. The MR can be determined by oxygen energy equivalents.

The basal metabolic rate (BMR) is minimal level of calories needed to sustain life.

The process of fat thermogenisis plays only a small role in calorie-burning in the average adult. The high level of sympathetic stimulation needed to produce it can be deleterious.

Exercise, or muscle activity, is the best way to burn calories. The muscles must contract against a load for maximal effect.

That some athletes are better at the strength events or the endurance events has a basis in physiology due to individual differences in the ratio of fast-twitch to slow-twitch muscle fibers.

Chapter 9 The Fasting State

After 8-10 hours of fasting, the body responds to low-normal glucose levels by shifting over to the burning of fats. This is orchestrated by several hormones

Hormones are molecules created by specialized cells or glands that are released into the bloodstream by a specific stimulus and act on specific cells for a specific effect. In this chapter we will look closely at insulin, glucagon, cortisol, growth hormone (GH), epinephrine, and norepinephrine — whose effects are similar to epinephrine.

Insulin

Insulin is a hormone of abundance. It is released not only by high carbohydrate levels — serum glucose — but also by high serum amino acid and free fatty acid levels.

Insulin is produced by the beta cells of the pancreas. The normal range of serum glucose is 70-90 mg/dl. Only when the level is over 90 mg/dl is insulin released. When the serum glucose rises over 100 mg/dl, insulin levels can quickly peak at 25 times baseline. Falling under 90 gm/dl, insulin secretion drops off just as fast, reaching very low levels within minutes.

Gly
Ile
Val
Glu
Gln
Phe
Cys
Cys   Ser   Leu
Val   Cys   Tyr   A chain
Asn   Thr
Gln   Ser   Ile
His   10
Leu   Gln
Cys   Leu
Gly   Glu
Ser   Asn
His   Tyr
10   Leu   Cys   21
Val   S
Glu   B chain   S
Ala   Cys   20
Leu   Tyr   Leu   Val   Gly
Thr
30   Lys
Pro
Thr
Tyr
Phe
Phe
Gly
Arg
Glu

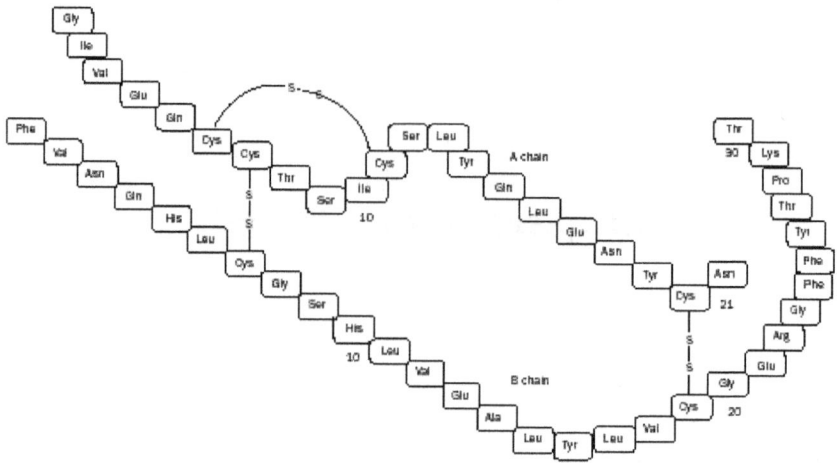

Above is an insulin molecule. Each square represents an amino acid joined in sequence by peptide bonds. Note that there are two amino acid chains, and three disulfide (S-S) bonds joining non-adjacent chain fragments.

Under the influence of insulin, excess carbohydrates are first stored as glycogen in the liver and muscles. When glycogen stores are sufficient, insulin acts to convert the carbohydrates into fat. This is eventually stored in either the liver or adipose tissue. Insulin also inhibits the breakdown of protein, fats, and glycogen.

Insulin has a short half-life and is cleared from the serum in about 12 minutes. This is important because a low glucose level can be just as deleterious as a high one. When activating a cell membrane receptor, insulin can increase the cell's rate of glucose uptake by 15 times baseline. Without insulin, there is minimal uptake of glucose by almost all the cells of the body — except for the brain cells which are freely permeable to it. Brain neurons use glucose exclusively for fuel under normal conditions.

Insulin and Glucagon

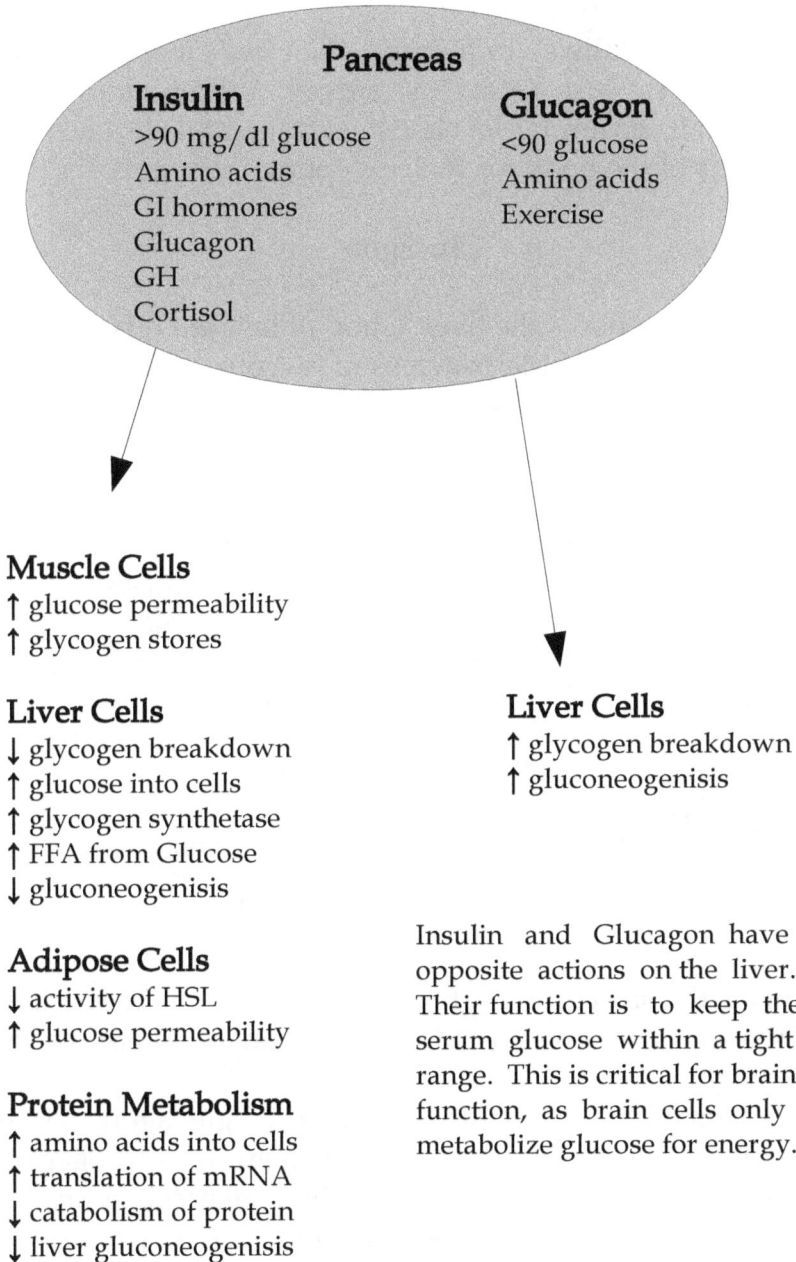

Pancreas

Insulin
>90 mg/dl glucose
Amino acids
GI hormones
Glucagon
GH
Cortisol

Glucagon
<90 glucose
Amino acids
Exercise

Muscle Cells
↑ glucose permeability
↑ glycogen stores

Liver Cells
↓ glycogen breakdown
↑ glucose into cells
↑ glycogen synthetase
↑ FFA from Glucose
↓ gluconeogenisis

Adipose Cells
↓ activity of HSL
↑ glucose permeability

Protein Metabolism
↑ amino acids into cells
↑ translation of mRNA
↓ catabolism of protein
↓ liver gluconeogenisis

Liver Cells
↑ glycogen breakdown
↑ gluconeogenisis

Insulin and Glucagon have opposite actions on the liver. Their function is to keep the serum glucose within a tight range. This is critical for brain function, as brain cells only metabolize glucose for energy.

Insulin also facilitates entry of specific amino acids into the cell and therefore is essential, along with growth hormone, for protein synthesis.

Without insulin's influence, the body's metabolism defaults to the use of fat for energy. Within minutes of insulin's fall, serum fat levels rise and fat begins to be used by all cells of the body for fuel, excepting the brain cells.

Glucagon

Glucagon opposes the liver action of insulin. It is secreted by the alpha cells of the pancreas in response to low-normal blood sugar, less than 70 mg/dl.

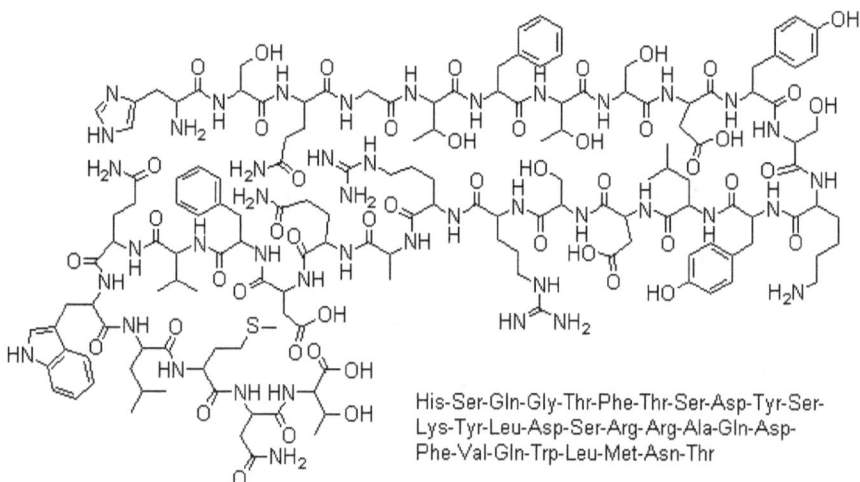

His-Ser-Gln-Gly-Thr-Phe-Thr-Ser-Asp-Tyr-Ser-Lys-Tyr-Leu-Asp-Ser-Arg-Arg-Ala-Gln-Asp-Phe-Val-Gln-Trp-Leu-Met-Asn-Thr

This is the structure of glucagon, with the chain of amino acids expanded — the specific amino acid sequence on the lower right.

The immediate effect of the release of glucagon, within minutes, is to promote the breakdown of glycogen to glucose in the liver, which is then released into the bloodstream. Glucagon also facilitates the process of

86 The Essene Diet

gluconeogenisis, where glucose is synthesized *de novo* in the liver from amino acids. By indirectly stimulating the production of specific enzymes, glucagon also causes the liver to take up amino acids from the serum.

Both insulin and glucagon can be thought of as two arms of a quick-response system for the purposes of maintaining the glucose level between 70- 90 mg/dl. The liver serves as a buffer organ for this crucial function. When the glucose is high, insulin causes the liver to become a "sink" and convert   excess glucose into glycogen and fat. When glucose levels are low, glucagon causes the liver to become a "source" of glucose through first the breakdown of glycogen, and then the synthesis glucose from amino acids.

Cortisol

Cortisol is synthesized from cholesterol. Note the 4-ring base cyclic structure from the cholesterol precursor.

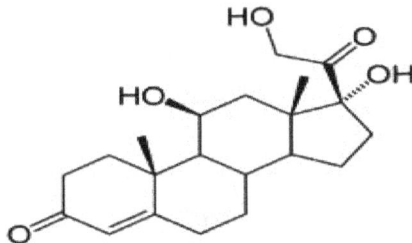

Cortisol synthesis and release from the cortex of the adrenal gland is caused by another hormone, ACTH, or adrenocorticotropin hormone, which is produced by the anterior pituitary gland. ACTH is released, in turn, by CRF or corticotropin releasing factor which is produced in the hypothalamus of the brain. Cortisol is produced when a

Cortisol and Epinephrine

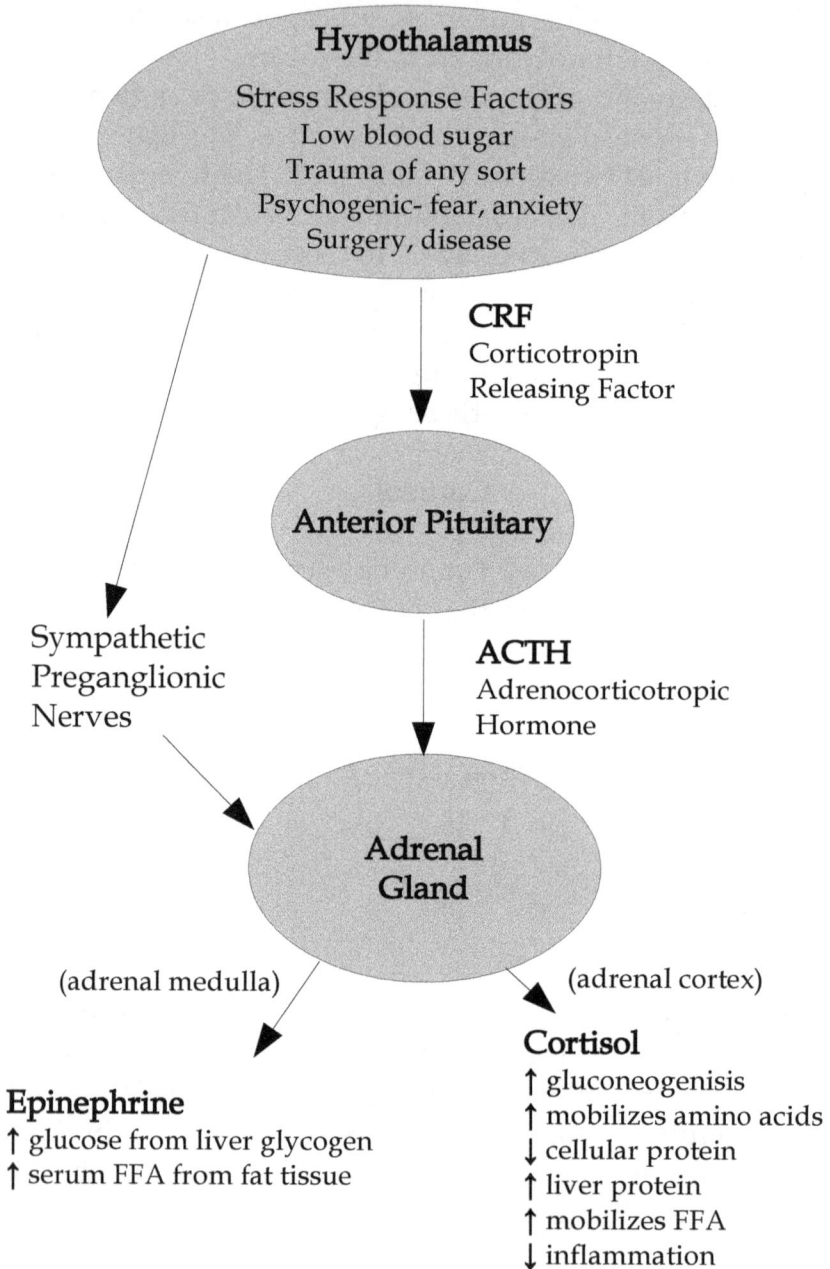

Hypothalamus

Stress Response Factors
Low blood sugar
Trauma of any sort
Psychogenic- fear, anxiety
Surgery, disease

CRF
Corticotropin
Releasing Factor

Anterior Pituitary

ACTH
Adrenocorticotropic
Hormone

Sympathetic
Preganglionic
Nerves

Adrenal Gland

(adrenal medulla)

(adrenal cortex)

Epinephrine
↑ glucose from liver glycogen
↑ serum FFA from fat tissue

Cortisol
↑ gluconeogenisis
↑ mobilizes amino acids
↓ cellular protein
↑ liver protein
↑ mobilizes FFA
↓ inflammation

88 The Essene Diet

stressful situation is identified by the hypothalamus — whether it is metabolic, traumatic, or psychogenic.

Cortisol is of a class of hormones called glucocorticoids. As the name suggests, it plays a key role in the mobilization of amino acids and some fats to enable the liver to make glucose through gluconeogenisis (glucose-new-origin). While glucagon also stimulates this process, the addition of cortisol can increase the rate of glucose production by 6 to 10 times.

In a fasting state lasting less than a week, cortisol mobilizes only "labile" proteins from cells. These are not basic functional proteins — such as contractile muscle or brain protein — but rather smooth muscle or enzyme protein. Also, the liver's production of protein is enhanced by the actions of cortisol, even while cortisol is causing labile proteins in the rest of the body to be broken down.

Cortisol also causes an increase in the storage of glycogen and has a delay effect in the body's use of glucose for energy — which is poorly understood. Possibly this is related to the need to spare serum glucose for use by the brain.

The overall effect of cortisol is to cause a rise in serum glucose to above normal levels which causes insulin to be released. Through an unknown mechanism, the presence of cortisol blunts the usual powerful effect of insulin on the uptake of glucose by the non-neural cell.

Cortisol has a similar mobilizing effect on adipose tissue, enhancing the release of fatty acids and glycerol into the blood. In the peripheral cells, it appears to have a direct positive effect on the oxidative metabolism of fats.

All of these actions helps the body shift from glucose to fat metabolism. The full effect, however, takes 2-3 hours to develop, compared with the rapid shift — within minutes — caused by the fall in insulin along with the rise in epinephrine.

The rapid response of cortisol to any type of stress suggests that it plays a significant role in survival. Possibly, the hypermetabolic state caused by disease and infection means that more glucose than normal is needed, or that raw amino acids are needed by the cell to repair damaged proteins rapidly.

Another important role that cortisol plays is as an anti-inflammatory agent. In many situations, such as allergic or asthmatic reactions, or viral or bacterial infections, the damage to the body is not done by the inciting event but rather the body's reaction to it. The mediators of inflammation produced by the cell — antibodies, prostaglandins, leukotrienes, lymphokines, etc. — can potentially have deadly results if they inadvertently attack the body. Rheumatoid Arthritis, for instance, is thought to be caused by an over-aggressive immune response to an infection, as is Systemic Lupus Erythmatosis and other "auto" immune diseases. Cortisol has a stabilizing effect on membranes of the cell organelles that make these mediators of inflammation, preventing their release.

Cortisol analogues have been proven to be life-saving in many situations for this reason. Prednisone has five times the strength of cortisol (hydrocortisone) on a per milligram basis, and dexamethasone has 15 times the potency. Artificial glucocorticoids have proven to be instrumental in organ transplants as they suppress the body's natural defense reaction to foreign tissue.

Growth Hormone

Growth Hormone (GH) is released from the anterior pituitary gland, located at the base of the brain, under the stimulus of growth hormone releasing factor (GHRF) which is produced by the ventromedial nucleus of the hypothalamus. This is the same hypothalamic nucleus that is sensitive to the serum glucose level and is crucial in the perception of satiety. Like cortisol, there is a large emotional-stress component to the release of GH. This is mediated through the hypothalamus.

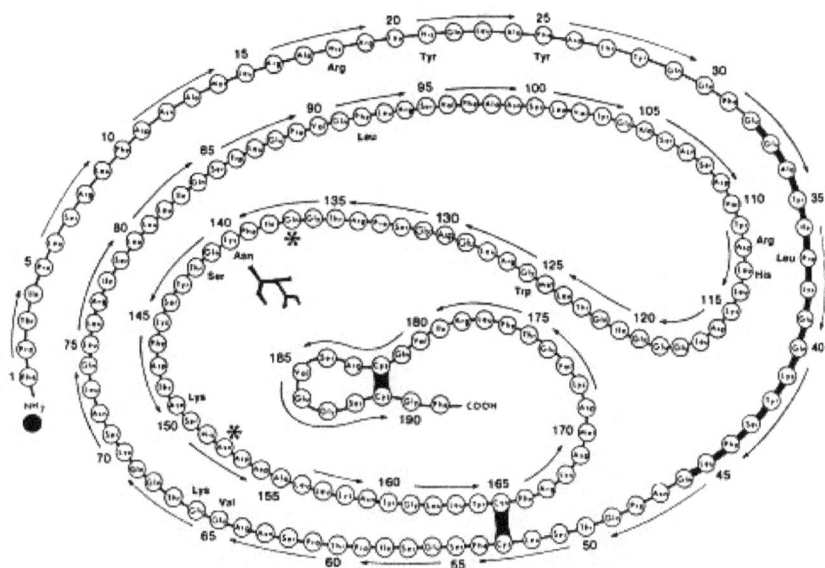

Growth hormone has protean effects throughout the body and is associated with energy abundance, as is insulin.

Growth Hormone

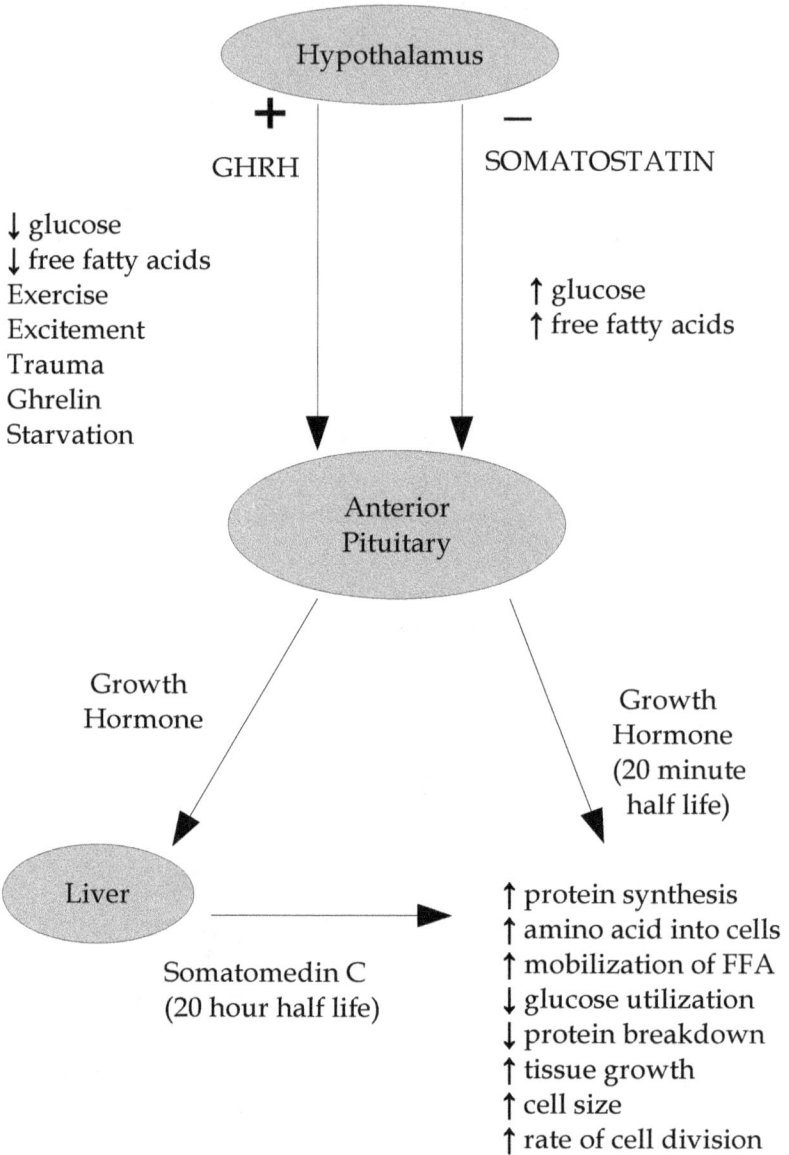

Hypothalamus

\+   −

GHRH   SOMATOSTATIN

↓ glucose
↓ free fatty acids
Exercise
Excitement
Trauma
Ghrelin
Starvation

↑ glucose
↑ free fatty acids

Anterior
Pituitary

Growth
Hormone

Growth
Hormone
(20 minute
half life)

Liver

Somatomedin C
(20 hour half life)

↑ protein synthesis
↑ amino acid into cells
↑ mobilization of FFA
↓ glucose utilization
↓ protein breakdown
↑ tissue growth
↑ cell size
↑ rate of cell division

Growth hormone stimulates growth in all cells that are capable of it, as well as cell division and differentiation. GH also affects energy metabolism. It increases production of proteins in the cell, mobilizes fatty acids from the adipose tissue for use in energy creation, and decreases the rate glucose utilization. In effect, growth hormone conserves or spares the body's use of carbohydrates.

Like insulin, GH facilitates the transport of amino acids into the cell. In fact, both GH and insulin are necessary for cell growth along with the presence of carbohydrates. Because of GH's effect on the mobilization of fats and their use as energy, GH also acts as a protein sparer as well as a carbohydrate sparer. So, over the long term, GH works on the body to promote the burning of fat and the production of muscle. The net result is an increase in lean body mass.

GH also functions as a counter to insulin, making tissues resistant to insulin's effects through an unknown mechanism.

While GH has a half-life of only 20 minutes in the serum, it causes secondary growth factors to be released. One of them, somatomedin C, has a half-life of 20 hours and is thought to be responsible for much of the effects usually attributed to growth hormone.

GH is secreted in pulsatile fashion, but the precise mechanism is unknown. Factors that stimulate release are starvation (related to ghrelin release in the stomach), low blood sugar and low serum fatty acids, exercise, excitement, and trauma. GH levels are also increased in the first few hours of sleep.

Epinephrine

Epinephrine is a neurotransmitter chemical that is released into the blood from sympathetic nerve endings in the adrenal medulla. Epinephrine is produced as a result of the activation of the hypothalamic "fight or flight" centers. It is also produced when the body is stressed through exercise.

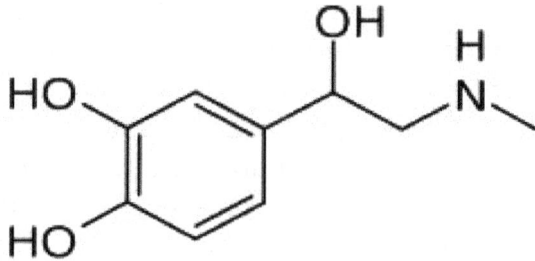

Epinephrine can be thought of as the serum messenger molecule of the sympathetic nervous system. In the blood, epinephrine can reach all of the cells of the body to exert its effects, whereas sympathetic nerves only reach certain target organs.

For the purposes of metabolism, epinephrine activates an enzyme in the adipose tissue, hormone sensitive lipase, that dramatically increases the release of free fatty acids into the blood — as high as eightfold within minutes of epinephrine's release. The fatty acids are then picked up by the muscle cells and used for fuel. A lesser effect of epinephrine is the breakdown of glycogen into glucose. It also stimulates thermogenisis in fat cells, discussed in the previous chapter.

Study Participants

With this information, answers can be hypothesized to explain the results reported by the pilot study participants. Scott wrote that while on the morning protocol he was able to lift more weight, and his muscle recovery time reverted to what it had been when he was a teenager 30 years previously.

The only way that muscles can get stronger is through gaining mass, i.e. the synthesis of more actin and myosin microfilaments. Also, the recovery time after a workout is partially dependent on the time it takes the body to repair muscle micro-trauma—always the goal of a "good" workout.

We know that during the morning fast, growth factors and cortisol levels are at maximal levels. The cortisol is mobilizing amino acids which are the building blocks of protein, although the primary goal is to use them for gluconeogenisis. GH and other growth factors are also at work, promoting specific amino acids to enter the body's cells. After the first meal at mid-day, insulin levels rise dramatically, stimulating other amino acids, as well as glucose, to enter the cell.

What can be hypothesized is that after the fast period is over, and the first meal consumed, a cellular metabolic "soup" is created that is optimal for the synthesis of muscle protein—growth factors, insulin, and a ready supply of amino acids. In this rich milieu, muscles grow and damaged proteins can be repaired relatively quickly.

The anti-inflammatory action of cortisol could also aid in the reduction of aches and pains felt after a workout which are due to the intentionally micro-damaged muscle tissue.

Mental Health Benefits

Participants reported feeling less "stressed out" while on the protocol. There is, in fact, a definite link between the affective mood disorders and levels of both cortisol and growth hormone, though the nature of the relationship has yet to be fully defined. Here, the anti-inflammatory and "pain killing" effect of cortisol could also be playing a role.

Daily Fast Physiology

Last meal ends at 9 p.m., awakening at 6 a.m.,
first meal at 11 a.m.

9 p.m.   GI hormones signal pancreas to release insulin. Blood
             glucose (BG) rises quickly. Insulin levels spike.
             Respiratory Quotient (RQ) approaches 1.0.

11   Carbohydrates and fats fully absorbed. Insulin levels
             remain high. Excess glucose converted to glycogen, fats

1 a.m.   Amino acids fully absorbed. RQ remains at 1.0.

4-5   Glucose stabilizes. Insulin falls. RQ at 1.0. Glycogen is
             broken down for glucose. Hunger contractions begin.

5-7   Liver glycogen levels fall. BS drops to 50-70 mg/dl.
             Low BS causes the release of glucagon, epinephrine.
             Insulin levels drop, metabolism shifts to burning fat.
             Hypothalamus releases CRF and GHRF with an
             increase in cortisol and GH. Cortisol mobilizes labile
             amino acids. RQ at .7.

7 a.m.   Cortisol levels 4 times normal. RQ remains at .7. GH
             causes synthesis of growth factors (somatomedin C).
             Gluconeogenisis begins.

9-11   Hunger contractions turn into pangs (first few days).
             Growth factors, cortisol levels high. RQ at .7.

11 a.m.   First meal. Insulin increases with blood sugar increase.
             Glucagon, cortisol, GH levels fall. GFs remain high.
             Metabolism shifts to carbohydrates. RQ returns to 1.0

A study out of England looked at the relationship between depression and growth hormone replacement in patients who were known to be GH deficient for various reasons.

Mahajan T, Crown A, et al; Atypical depression in growth hormone deficient adults, and the beneficial effects of growth hormone treatment on depression and quality of life; Eur J Endo (2004) 151 325–332

The study was small and lasted for only four months, but it was scientifically rigorous — being double-blinded and placebo controlled. Also, it was a cross-over study, which meant for the second half of it the placebo and GH groups were switched.

The abstract conclusion:

The results of our study confirm that a large proportion of GHDAs (growth hormone deficient adults) have unequivocal psychiatric morbidity, and suggest that a response to treatment can be seen after a short trial of GH therapy. We hypothesise that this rapid improvement of symptoms of atypical depression represents a direct central effect of GH therapy.

Does this translate over to normal adults? Certainly, GH levels tend to fall as people age. The extended fast period could serve to mitigate that decline, if not stop it altogether. Even with normal baseline levels of GH, an added "kick" — with the somatomedin C levels remaining high for up to a day or more — could go a long way in explaining the reduction in stress that all of the participants reported.

Added benefits of the morning fast!

Take Home Points

Insulin facilitates glucose entry into the cell. Insulin rises quickly when serum glucose levels are high, but falls just as quickly when serum glucose levels normalize.

Insulin and glucagon have opposite actions on the liver in maintaining serum glucose. The liver can be thought of as a glucose buffer organ, storing glucose when there is too much of it, and either releasing or creating glucose when there is too little of it.

Low-normal serum glucose levels triggers a "stress" response in the brain. Epinephrine, glucagon, cortisol, and growth hormone are released as a result.

The stress response can be caused by trauma, physiologic abnormalities, or psychogenic factors like fear.

Epinephrine causes the adipose tissue to release fats and encourages the breakdown of glycogen in the liver for glucose.

Glucagon also helps increase the liver breakdown of glycogen into glucose, and aids in gluconeogenisis.

Cortisol in the short-term facilitates the breakdown of labile proteins to amino acids which can be used in the making of glucose. Cortisol also helps the body shift over to fat metabolism, and it has anti-inflammatory and pain-killing properties as well.

Growth hormone stimulates the growth of the body's cells that are capable of it and facilitates the synthesis of protein. Growth hormone also might have mood-stabilizing effects.

Fat tissue, or adipose tissue, is in part an energy buffer organ. If too many calories are consumed, the excess will be stored as triglycerides and the adipose tissue will grow. If too few calories are ingested, triglycerides will be released for use and the adipose tissue will shrink.

Chapter 10 The Magic Bullet

Scientists have long been searching for a substance to blunt hunger—a "magic bullet" diet pill—with acceptable side effects. Modern researchers have narrowed their focus to brain neurotransmitters and hormone analogues. Today's sophisticated technology has allowed the identification of dozens of potential candidates. In fact, researchers are awash in bio-molecules that affect either appetite or satiety. No breakthroughs, however, can be seen on the horizon.

The Hypothalamus

The feeling of hunger is a formed from many different sensory inputs and modulated through the hypothalamus —a small area at the base of the thalamus in the brain's limbic system. There, neural centers for both appetite and satiety have been identified. The lateral area of the hypothalamus controls appetite, while satiety is controlled in the ventromedial nucleus. This has been determined through countless rat brain oblation/stimulation studies.

The limbic system of the brain got its name because the structures that compose it border the base of the cerebral cortices. It is in this system where the vegetative functions of the body are controlled and where emotions and motivational drive originate.

Neural-Hormonal Control of Hunger

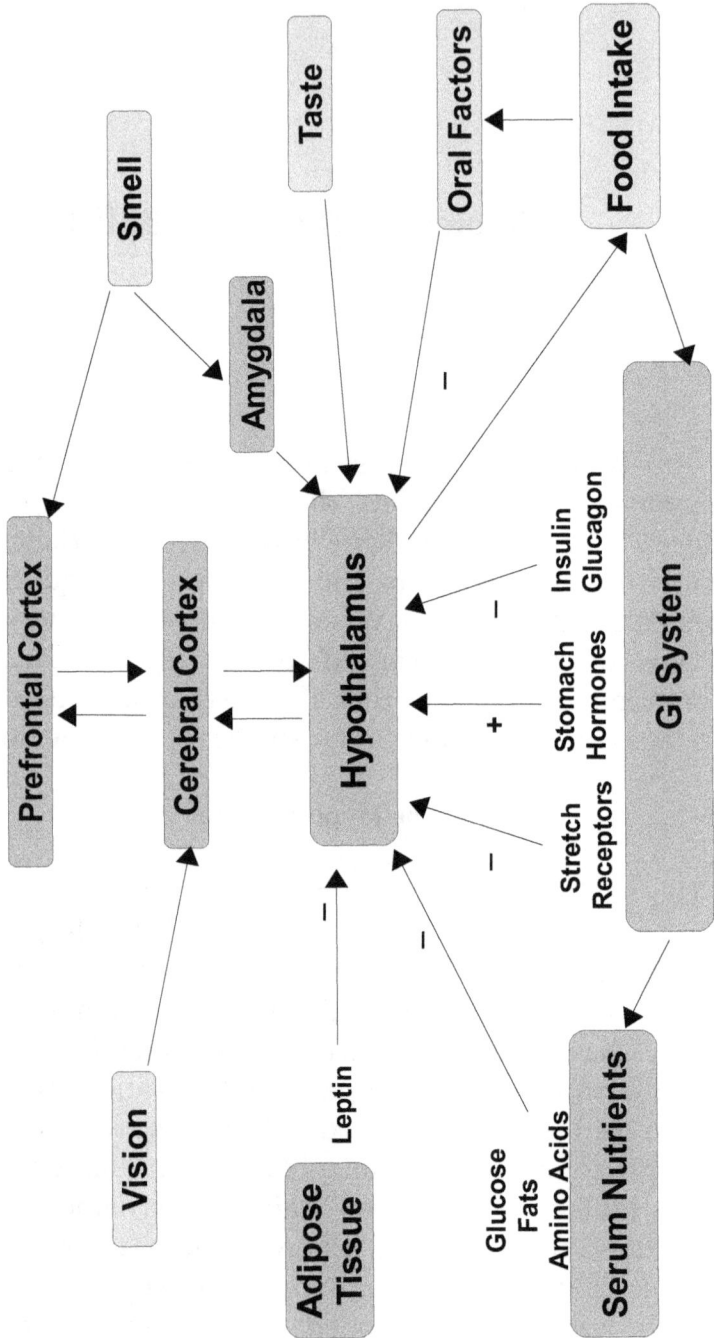

blood that regulate energy balance and metabolism. The pancreas, part of the digestive system, also releases hormones that effect these parameters, such as insulin, glucagon, and somatostatin, as do secretions from the adrenal and pituitary glands.

The chart on the opposing page shows how the appetite and satiety centers in the hypothalamus are modified by various inputs. Of note are the connections from the cerebral and pre-frontal cortices – the centers of higher thought and executive action –, as well as afferent pathways from the rest of the body. The cerebral cortices are assumed to be the most recently evolved structure of the brain. Usually the cortices serve an inhibitory function over the more reactionary limbic system – the so-called reptilian brain. Interestingly, sight and smell feed into the hypothalamus directly from these higher cortical areas.

The sense of smell, or olfaction, plays a large role in the perception of hunger. It is the oldest of the sensations from an evolutionary standpoint, but it has evolved two more "layers" over tens of millions of years. The newest of these smell centers connects the olfactory receptors in the nose directly to the paleocortex of the amygdala, bypassing the lower limbic system completely.

Sight is mediated in the occipital cortex which sends fibers to the limbic system and the hypothalamus. Taste first is processed in the thalamus, and then has connections to the cerebral cortex. The physical act of feeding is coordinated by a collection of very primitive reflex arcs originating in the midbrain. When activated, this area sends inhibitory signals back to the hypothalamus to avoid over-eating. Also when the stomach engorges with food, the smooth muscle stretch receptors send inhibitory signals to the hypothalamus.

Magic Bullet Candidates

Modern researchers have identified many "magic bullet" candidates. While all of these substances play a role, none of them appears to play a dominant role — excepting for a class of drugs to be discussed later. To illustrate the complexity of the appetite/satiety system, these substances that scientists have isolated and evaluated as having promise are listed. Orexigenic substances are those that stimulate the appetite and so must be blocked. Anorexigenic substances reduce the appetite and so must be stimulated or analogues formulated.

Orexigenic Neurotransmitters and Hormones

Neuropeptide Y - a 36-amino acid neurotransmitter that is produced in the hypothalamus. The substance increases the urge to feed and increases the amount of energy stored as fat.

Melanin Concentrating Hormone – a 19-amino acid compound produced in the hypothalamus that increases food intake and weight gain when administered centrally. It also influences mood and the sleep-wake cycle.

Orexins A and B - a group of neurotransmitters produced in the hypothalamus that stimulates appetite and is crucial in arousal-awakefulness functions of the brain.

Endorphins - opiate-like substances produced in the hypothalamus and pituitary gland that, among many other functions, stimulate the hunger for spicy food (!).

Galanin - a neuropeptide widely found in the central nervous system. Galanin plays a poorly understood role in many processes, including the stimulation of hunger.

Glutamate - excitetory neurotransmitter that also serves as a non-essential amino acid. It plays a role in many brain processes, including a poorly understood one in the stimulation of appetite.

Cortisol - steroid hormone produced by the adrenal cortex. It increases the feeding impulse and encourages the body to convert fats and amino acids into glucose.

Ghrelin - hormone produced by the stomach in the fasting state. It stimulates the hypothalamus to produce NPY to increase the desire to consume high calorie food.

Endocannaboids- - neuro-modulatory lipids that affect brain areas involved in appetite, pain sensations, motor learning, and other functions. The effect of marijuana is mediated through this substance.

Anorexigenic Substances

Cocaine- and ampetamine-regulated transcript (CART)- produced in the arcuate nucleus of the hypothalamus and suppresses the appetite.

Serotonin - a neurotransmitter that is also found in large quantities in the gut where it regulates intestinal movements (peristalsis). In the brain, it helps regulate mood, sleep, and appetite where it has a mild inhibitory effect.

Norepinephrine – a catecholamine that serves as a neurotransmitter as well as a hormone. It is released with sympathetic stimulation and suppresses feelings of hunger as part of the flight-or-flight response to stress.

Alpha Melanocyte Stimulating Hormone - a peptide hormone produced by the pituitary gland. Studies indicate it inhibits food consumption.

Corticotropin Releasing Hormone (CRH) – a stress hormone produced in the hypothalamus. It decreases feeding in mice studies.

Insulin - is produced by the beta-cells of the pancreas; it has an appetite suppressant effect on the brain.

Cholecystokinin - is produced in the duodenum in response to fats, suppresses appetite by a poorly-understood mechanism, but thought to be peripheral rather than central.

Glucagon-like Peptide – an intestinal peptide that increases satiety in the brain by an unknown mechanism.

Leptin – a protein hormone produced in adipose tissue and acts on the hypothalamus to decrease fat storage.

An extensive list, indeed.

Remember, too, that depending on the type of action a substance might have, the scientist must explore ways to make an analogue to it, or imitate a substance that naturally increases the substance's levels, or that blocks its destruction. Additionally, every substance acts upon a specific cell receptor for its effect, so the receptor itself might be blocked, or "beefed up" to increase or decrease the effect of the substance as the case may be.

Then, after overcoming these preliminary research hurdles and defining a testable "magic bullet" substance, long and expensive clinical trials must begin—most of which prove to be disappointments.

Leptin and Ghrelin

For example, leptin and ghrelin initially held promise, but their efficacy was not confirmed by clinically.

Leptin is produced by the body's adipose tissue at levels corresponding to the adipose tissue mass. In people with normal weight, high leptin levels serve to decrease appetite —apparently a negative feedback mechanism put into play when fat stores are excessive. If a leptin analogue could be made in pill form, theoretically the appetite centers would be depressed, or the satiety centers stimulated.

However, further research revealed that obese people have high levels of leptin in their serum, but their appetite is unaffected. The scientists then turned their attention to the leptin receptors in the hypothalamus of their obese subjects, but those receptors were found to be normal. For whatever reason, the inescapable conclusion was that the leptin anorexic effect works only in people who have relatively normal levels of fat stores to begin with.

Likewise, studies into the "hunger" hormone ghrelin have been disappointing. Ghrelin is produced by the stomach in the starvation mode. Studies have shown that it intensifies the urge to consume high-calorie carbohydrates and fats, mediated through the hypothalamus and neuropeptide NPY. If ghrelin could be blocked or the ghrelin receptors in the hypothalamus inactivated, the hunger urge might be squelched. But, like leptin, further studies demonstrated that in obese individuals the effects of increasing ghrelin levels were minimal.

The Sympathetic Nervous System

There is a class of pharmaceuticals, however, that successfully suppresses appetite, but they have adverse side effects. FDA approval of them is for only short-term use. These drugs stimulate the sympathetic nervous system. The illegal drug amphetamine is of this class.

The human sympathetic nervous system (SNS) is a part of the autonomic nervous system (ANS). The SNS is not under direct volitional control, and is designed prepare us for immediate action when a dangerous situation is perceived. The initiating stress can be psychologically generated, as in fear, or physically-driven, as in trauma or severe blood loss.

When the SNS is stimulated, drastic effects are seen as the body readies itself for extreme physical exertion — either to fight or to run away. Through the selective constriction or dilatation of circulatory vessels, blood is shunted away from the digestive tract and concentrated in the heart, muscles, and lungs. The heart rate also increases along with the force of the heart's contraction. Stress hormones such as cortisol, epinephrine, and norepinephrine are released.

Of special interest to the individual seeking to lose weight, under SNS stimulation the appetite centers of the hypothalamus are virtually shut down. Also, calories are burned as the metabolic rate increases.

Parasympathetic Nervous System

The ANS has a counter arm to the SNS called the parasympathetic nervous system (PNS). When the parasympathetic system is stimulated (through the Vagus nerve) the heart rate slows, the blood pressure normalizes, and blood is delivered to the digestive system at the expense of the voluntary musculature. Conditions that are ripe for growth and reproduction are created, and the appetite returns.

An easy way to remember the two arms of the ANS is "sympathetic-survival, parasympathetic-peace."

Autonomic Nervous System

Organ	Sympathetic	Parasympathetic
Heart	↑ rate, force	↓ rate
Blood Vessels	constriction	no effect
Lung Bronchi	dilated	constricted
Gut Lumen	↓ peristalsis	↑ peristalsis
Liver	↑ glucose	↑ glycogen
Kidney	↓ urine output	no effect
Appetite	decreased	no effect
Blood	↑ glucose, lipids	no effect
BMR	↑ up to 100%	no effect
Skeletal Muscle	↑ strength	no effect
Mental activity	increased	no effect
Fat cells	lipolysis (thermal?)	no effect
Pupil	dilated	constricted
Pancreas Glands	↑ secretion	↑ secretion

Side Effects

Sympathetic drugs are successful in suppressing the appetite and weight is lost. But the side effects are considerable and potentially disastrous — such as a rapid heart rate, high blood pressure, nervousness, and sleeplessness. Scientists are continuing to work on a more selective drug of this class.

The stimulation of the sympathetic system is also needed for the thermogenisis property of fat to take effect. This was discussed in a previous chapter. The effect, if clinical trials are confirmatory, would be small for the amount of sympathetic stimulus needed.

Currently, several drugs of the sympathetic class have been approved for short-term use only. Long-term clinical trials have shown that the dramatic weight loss achieved initially usually fades over time as the individual becomes tolerant to the drug. Sustained weight loss of no more than 15% is possible—and at the cost of significant cardiovascular side effects.

Serotonin Agonists

Serotonin is a neurotransmitter known to have an inhibitory effect on neural pain pathways in the central nervous system (CNS), which includes the brain and spinal cord. Serotonin also helps to control mood, impulsive behavior, and obsessionality. Serotonin agonists play a major role, along with other psychotropic drugs, in most of the major psychiatric disorders, including disorders of thought (schizophrenia) and disorders of mood (depression and anxiety).

It is speculated that stimulating the formation of serotonin or blocking its destruction (thereby prolonging its effect) has a modulating effect on the feeling of fullness and satiety. While these serotonin-like drugs have been linked to weight loss in clinical trials, a causal relationship has not been established. The weight loss in any case is marginal.

The serotonin agonists have had a stormy history. The effects of serotonin are system-wide and not yet fully understood. The early FDA-approved serotonin-like drugs, fenfluramine and dexfenfluramine, were found to also stimulate the serotonin receptors on cardiac valvular tissue and pulmonary arterial musculature, causing pulmonary hypertension (PHT). Both serotonin agonists were removed from the market.

Recently, the FDA approved lorcaserin, a selective serotonin agonist, for use in conjunction with diet and exercise as an effective tool for weight loss. Lorcaserin experimentally has a very low affinity for the cardiac and pulmonary serotonin receptors. However, the FDA specifically declined to affirm the cardiovascular safety of lorcaserin long-term. Clinical studies involving lorcaserin used by the FDA lasted for only two years (as of this writing in September 2012). It took five years on average for the PHT to develop in people taking fenfluramine or dexfenfluramine.

Though there is a huge psychogenic-psychiatric component to eating and weight gain, broad generalities cannot be made. Depression can produce either weight gain or weight loss depending on the individual, as can anxiety and other disturbances of mood.

Lipase Blockers

There is another "magic bullet" pill that can virtually guarantee weight loss if used consistently. It does not work on the hypothalamus and feeding centers of the brain, and it does not effect hunger. The drug orlistat neutralizes gastric and pancreatic lipase in the gut lumen. Without the means to break down the lipids ingested, much of the fats are passed through the digestive tract and excreted unabsorbed. While effective, orlistat causes flatulence and other socially unpleasant gastrointestinal side effects. It is not a popular weight loss option.

Take Home Points

Hunger and appetite are effected by multiple and redundant neural pathways which themselves are subject to many positive and negative feedback loops. Slaying the "beast" of hunger is like battling a 70-headed hydra. Blocking only one pathway, or even two or three, is ineffective as other pathways come to the fore.

Weight can be lost through the activation of the sympathetic nervous system, but the side effects are undesirable. Lipase-blocking drugs also have undesirable side effects.

Mood-stabilizing drugs have not shown consistent weight loss effects when the exercise factor is removed.

This ends our journey into physiology and metabolics — a complicated world, indeed!

As promised, we will now look at the evidence presented by the two biggest breakfast food companies in support of their ad campaigns.

Chapter 11 Kellogg's

Kellogg's tackles the breakfast issue head-on on their corporate web site "Kelloggs.com." The conclusion is not surprising—adults need their breakfast!

> Even as adults, the benefits of breakfast can be significant. Not only do breakfast eaters get more nutrients, they eat fewer calories and less fat and cholesterol then those who don't eat breakfast...Plus, adults who regularly enjoy breakfast tend to have healthier body weights and are more physically active than those who pass up the meal.

The paragraph is footnoted, so we can look at the studies that support their statements. The first two sentences share a single reference: a 2007 article in the Nutrition Review journal.

> Timlin MT, Pereira MA. *Breakfast frequency and quality in the etiology of adult obesity and chronic diseases.* Nutr Rev. 2007;65:268-281.

The Timlin study's abstract, however, is NOT supportive of what Kellogg's states.

> Many observational studies have found that breakfast frequency is inversely associated with obesity and chronic disease, but this literature does have some important

limitations. Only four relatively small and short-term randomized trials have examined breakfast consumption and body weight or chronic disease risk, with mixed results. Large, long-term, randomized trials are needed.

The Timlin study is a review study, meaning that it looks at dozens of other studies and draws conclusions based upon them. For Kellogg's to reference a review article for such targeted assertions should not be acceptable. If there were specific nutritional studies that unequivocally supported Kellogg's two statements rest assured they would have been cited.

Let us take a closer look the first part of the Kellogg's statements.

Even as adults, the benefits of breakfast can be significant.

Note the waffle-wording. The benefits of breakfast "can be significant," and not "*are* significant."

And even if, for the sake of argument, it is assumed that over time breakfast eaters get more nutrients, eat less calories, less fat, and consume less cholesterol than breakfast skippers, does that make any difference in real world health outcomes? Prospective clinical trials are needed, as the Timlin abstract recommends.

The second part of Kellogg's assertion makes claims regarding adults and breakfast.

Plus, adults who regularly enjoy breakfast tend to have healthier body weights and are more physically active than those who pass up the meal.

An obvious problem is seen. People who are more physically active will, of course, tend to have "healthier" body weights whether they eat breakfast or not, as they will burn off more calories. Note the waffle-word "tend." Kellogg's doesn't outright declare a causal relationship between the eating of breakfast and a healthier body weight because it can't. The eating of breakfast could very well just be a part of a lifestyle set for these individuals — a set which includes regular exercise.

Kellogg's, however, references four studies in support of the statement. The first is out of Massachusetts:

> Ma Y et al. *Association between eating patterns and obesity in a free-living US adult population.* Am J Epidemiol. 2003;158:85-92.

The Ma study enrolled 499 people and followed them for a year. Five times during the year, the subjects completed a 24-hour recall for three days regarding their eating habits and exercise levels. Weights and other variables were also determined at that time. The self-reported diet data was then interpolated for the entire year. If a participant reported not eating a breakfast 75% of the time, they were included in the breakfast-skipping group.

The researchers found that the breakfast-skipping group was 4.5 times more likely to be obese than those who ate breakfast. Outwardly, this is an impressive number. But there are some problems with the study that the researchers themselves acknowledge.

The number in the breakfast-skipping group was very small, only 3.5% of the 499 person total — or about 18 individuals. This percentage is far lower than the accepted 25% estimated national average for breakfast-skipping. The study authors admitted that the "4.5 times" figure was of questionable significance.

They then rejiggered the numbers and included in the breakfast-skipping group anyone who reported missing at least one breakfast in any of the 15 days of self-reported diet data.

The percentage of breakfast-skippers then went up to 27% with the likelihood of obesity dropping precipitously from 4.5 times to 1.34 times normal.

The Ma study also kept data on the physical activity level of all of its participants. This factor was used in their multivariate analysis, but not reported independently. How would that correlate with the reported data in the breakfast-skipping group? We need to know.

As with many clinical studies of this nature, there was a large drop-out rate. Of the 1254 individuals who met the enrollment requirements, 641 entered into the protocol with only 267 subjects completing the entire year. The researchers, desperate to gain statistical power, included in the final results those who completed at least 10 of the 15 dietary recalls to make the number of participants 499.

Another confounding variable, among others, was that only a single year's data was collected. As the authors conclude:

> Although we found that eating patterns were associated with obesity, the findings cannot be considered causal. For example, current diet may not be representative of diet in previous years (which is the diet that led to obesity, not the current diet).

Key passage — "...the findings cannot be considered causal."

The second study Kellogg's references is an analysis of the data from the National Health survey (1988-91, 1991-94), with 16,000 people included in the data analysis:

Cho S et al. *The effect of breakfast type on total daily energy intake and Body Mass Index: Results from the Third National*

Health and Nutrition Examination Survey (NHANES III). J Am Coll Nutr. 2003;22:296-302.

In this benchmark and oft-referenced study, a full 20% of the participants were breakfast-skippers, on par with the national average. Interestingly, subgroups were delineated made up of those who ate specific types of breakfasts — cold cereals (ready-to-eat cereal or RTEC), cooked cereals, eggs and bacon, dairy products — as well as those who skipped breakfast entirely. A body mass index (BMI) was independently determined for all of these participants and 24 hour diet recalls were obtained, along with other data.

The results showed that the average breakfast skipper had a BMI of 26.92 while the average cold cereal eater had an BMI of 26.03 — a difference of just under five pounds. This, however, compares to an INCREASE in the BMI at 27.04 in the average meat-and-eggs breakfast eater, and an increase at 27.11 in the average dairy product breakfast eater. The lowest BMI average was the cooked cereal breakfast eater with a BMI of 25.41.

Admittedly, this is a "win" of sorts for the cereal giants, but not for the eating of breakfast as a whole. The Kellogg's statement that "adults who regularly enjoy breakfast tend to have healthier body weights" only applies to those who consume certain types of breakfasts.

Of more interest, and not brought up by Kellogg's, is that the Cho study found breakfast skippers consumed 10% LESS daily calories on average than did the RTEC breakfast eaters. This begs the question: if breakfast skippers consume less calories per day than RTEC breakfast consumers, then why is their BMI slightly greater?

The Cho study authors advanced a convoluted theory as to why this significant result was found.

However, we found that the skippers have the lowest total daily energy intake of all groups, despite having high BMIs. An explanation for this could be that subjects who skip breakfast are already overweight, are trying to lose weight and are also limiting their daily energy intake from other food sources throughout the day. From these data it cannot be determined whether the association is causal (skipping breakfast leading to poor dietary patterns leading to obesity) or correlational (persons who skip breakfast are already overweight and are trying to control it by skipping breakfast). In either case, it is clear from these and other data that skipping breakfast does not lead to attaining or maintaining a healthy weight.

In the last sentence, the Cho group doggedly sticks to their belief in the myth of breakfast despite their own study's evidence to the contrary. Cho simply ignores the obvious: People fastidious about breakfast are probably also fastidious about regular exercise and other health issues. Controlling for exercise, which this study claims to have done, is very unreliable given that the data is self-reported.

The third reference is an epidemiologic study as well:

Song WO et al. *Is consumption of breakfast associated with body mass index in US adults?* J Am Diet Assoc. 2005;105:1373-1382.

The study is an analysis of data from the National Health and Nutrition Examination Survey of 1999-2000. It included 4,218 men and women. Breakfast-skippers were not included.

The purpose of the study was to see if types of breakfasts could predict BMI. The researchers found:

RTEC breakfast consumption...predicted weight status in women, but not in men.

But why the disparity? Before the breakfast food companies can cite this study with any gusto, the difference must be explained. The result must be considered spurious.

From the study abstract:

...the effects of physiological variables and health-related behaviors on the relationship between total and RTEC intake at breakfast and weight status, remain to be established.

The fourth referenced study is a twin-parent study out of Finland:

Keski-Rahkonen A et al. *Breakfast skipping and health-compromising behaviors in adolescents and adults.* Eur J Clin Nutr. 2003;57.

Self-reported data from twin sets and their parents in a specific time period were obtained and analyzed, along with corresponding health records. Regarding the adults, the researchers reported:

...smoking, infrequent exercise, low education level, male sex, higher BMI, and more frequent alcohol use were associated with breakfast skipping.

The study links breakfast skipping in adults with a significantly higher BMI, but it also links breakfast skipping to infrequent exercise. Clearly, the cause of a higher BMI in adults could easily, and probably, be the lack of exercise, and not the skipping of breakfast.

Moving on to Kellogg's promotional website "Ready to Eat," another referenced statement is found.

Research shows that regular breakfast-eaters, both adults and kids, tend to have healthier body weights than breakfast skippers. Those who eat breakfast also tend to make healthier food choices throughout the day .

For the first sentence, an Australian study is cited:

Smith KJ et al. *Skipping breakfast: longitudinal associations with cardiometabolic risk factors in the Childhood Determinants of Adult Health Study*. J Am Diet Assoc. 2010.

It looked at children and adolescents (ages 9-15) who were initially interviewed in 1985 about their eating habits. Body measurements were taken along with blood drawn to determine baseline serum markers. These same individuals were interviewed 20 years later as adults and the tests and measurements were repeated.

The point of the study was to determine how the eating or skipping of breakfast affected serum and weight-related cardiometabolic risk factors. One factor considered was abdominal girth, a significant predictor of future cardiovascular disease.

To analyze the data, the researchers divided the individuals into four groups: 1) those who ate breakfast regularly as children and later as adults, 2) those who ate breakfast only as children and not as adults, 3) those who ate breakfast only as adults and not children, and 4) those who skipped breakfast both as children and adults.

The results demonstrated that the group that skipped breakfast as both children and adults tended to have a greater waist circumference, higher LDL cholesterol levels, and higher fasting insulin levels than those who ate breakfast both as children and adults. On the surface, this would tend to support Kellogg's assertion that both adults and children benefited from breakfast.

However, Kellogg's ignored group 2—those who ate breakfast as a child but skipped breakfast as adults. A control group! As the Essene Diet protocol is intended for adults only, and children are encouraged to eat breakfast, this is very significant.

In group 2, the adult BMI profiles were almost identical to group 1, where adults ate breakfast both as adults and children. The obesity rate (BMI over 30) was 17% in the former, compared to 14% in the latter. Also, both groups had almost identical rates of abdominal obesity, at 32%.

Considering those results, Kellogg's statement is not supported — rather the opposite.

In group 4, those who did not eat breakfast either as children or adults, the obesity rate was 28%, nearly double. As expected, the abdominal obesity rate was also higher, at 43%.

The study suggests only that skipping breakfast as a child is unhealthy — which no one would disagree with. For the individual who skips breakfast as an adult after eating breakfast as a child, the study identifies no significant increase in cardiometabolic risk factors.

The study authors conclude:

> Participants who skipped breakfast in adulthood but not in childhood had meal patterns similar to those who skipped breakfast at both time points. However, participants who skipped breakfast at both time points were the only group to have had a significantly larger waist circumference and higher cardiometabolic risk factors than those who ate breakfast at both time points.

Let us move on to the second sentence in the paragraph on the "Ready to Eat" site.

> Those who eat breakfast also tend to make healthier food choices throughout the day.

Exactly who "those" is referring to is unclear, but from the previous sentence, it will be taken to mean both adults and children. Do adults make healthier food choices throughout the day if they eat breakfast?

The first reference is to a review study:

Rampersaud GC, Pereira MA, Girard BL, Adams J, Metzl JD. *Breakfast habits, nutritional status, body weight, and academic performance in children and adolescents*. J Am Diet Assoc. 2005;105:743-760

The study abstract, however, refers only to children and adolescents, and not adults. Even then, the study conclusions were lukewarm at best:

Although the quality of breakfast was variable within and between studies, children who reported eating breakfast on a consistent basis tended to have superior nutritional profiles than their breakfast-skipping peers. Breakfast eaters generally consumed more daily calories yet were less likely to be overweight, although not all studies associated breakfast skipping with overweight.

What does a superior nutritional profile mean? How does it translate into real world health benefits? Kellogg's suggests that it does, but provides no prospective studies to support it. Interestingly, those children who skipped breakfast consumed less calories during the day, but had a higher BMI — results reminiscent of the Cho study.

The second referenced study is the Keski-Rahkonen study out of Finland, which we have previously discussed.

Also on the Kellogg's "Ready to Eat" web site is a PDF document put out by its Canadian marketing branch. The intriguing title is "Breakfast: A Tool in Weight Management."

This deserves a closer look!

> ...Yet compelling research on breakfast eaters and skippers suggests that breakfast may be a useful tool in weight management, and so developing strategies to help Canadians overcome existing barriers to eating breakfast are important.

"Compelling" is even more of an obfuscatory waffle word than "linked" or "suggested." It hints of a great natural truth that the researchers are just on the verge of discovering.

Several statements follow in the colorful brochure that are not only referenced, but the references themselves are discussed. Among them we find our old friends — studies put out by Cho, Song, Ma, and Keski-Rahkonen.

> Numerous studies have examined the relationship between breakfast consumption and body weight and/or body mass index (BMI). Most studies have shown that breakfast eaters tend to have lower BMIs than breakfast skippers.

The Cho study is discussed first.

> Cho and colleagues analysed the dietary recall records of 16,452 adults from NHANES III (1988-1994) and found that men and women who ate breakfast had significantly lower BMIs than breakfast skippers after controlling for age, gender, race, smoking, alcohol intake, physical activity and poverty index.

If we parse the study by types of breakfasts consumed, the first statement is false. The Cho study showed that only those who ate cooked or ready-to-eat cereal had lower BMIs than those who skipped breakfast. Those who ate breakfasts of eggs, meat, or dairy products had a HIGHER BMI than those who skipped breakfast.

Next, the Song study is discussed.

> Another trial using NHANES data (1999-2000, n=218) conducted by Song and colleagues compared breakfast and BMI in men and women. After adjusting for various obesity-related covariates, results showed that women who skipped breakfast were more likely to have a BMI of 25 or greater (OR=0.76, 95% confidence interval: 0.57-1.01). However, when cereal intake at breakfast was added as a covariate to the analysis, the significant association between breakfast and BMI disappeared. This study also addressed breakfast type by classifying data as RTEC breakfast and non-RTEC breakfast. Here, RTEC breakfast consumption had a significant inverse relationship with BMI in women after adjusting for the same covariates (OR=0.70, 95% confidence interval: 0.52-0.94).

As we previously observed, if the RTEC breakfast were so globally beneficial, men should be affected as well as women. Why aren't they? There are other factors at work.
On to the Ma study:

> Ma and colleagues examined the association between breakfast skipping and BMI in 499 adults. Subjects were followed for one year and an average 13.4 dietary recall records and 4.8 BMI calculations were collected per person. Results showed that breakfast skippers were 4.5 times more likely to be obese (BMI>30) than breakfast eaters (95% confidence interval: 1.57–12.90).

As we have also discussed, the obesity number is very misleading, as admitted to by the study's authors. The study had a high drop-out rate with selection and "stay in" bias. The breakfast skippers made up less than four percent of the total — 18 people in all — and etc etc etc.

The Keski-Rahkonen report was discussed, but only to support the importance of breakfast in children and adolescence, which we do not question.

Further on in the PDF brochure:

> Evidence suggests that people who eat breakfast are slimmer than breakfast skippers; although the findings are not always consistent.

This is very misleading, and note the waffle word "suggests." The use of "not always" would be more accurate if "always" was dropped. And we have to return to the 16,000 participant Cho study where it was found that people who eat a non-cereal breakfast have a higher BMI than those who skip breakfast.

> Some researchers have suggested that treating all breakfasts alike may confound results and that the type of food eaten at breakfast may be an important determinant. As shown in the study by Song and colleagues, RTEC breakfast consumption more strongly predicted BMI than breakfast of any type.

The Song study certainly gives the cereal companies some grist to chew on; there is a defensible relationship between the eating of cereal and a lower BMI. We have talked about the lifestyle factor in explaining those numbers.

It might also be the case that in filling up one's stomach with low-calorie cereal, one is NOT filling up their stomach with higher calorie meat, eggs, and dairy products. If that is the case, then eating cereal at lunch or dinner would probably give the same BMI improvement — as slight as it is (7-10 pounds). But don't expect the cereal giants to initiate studies to investigate this.

Another statement:

> More generally, reviews of studies of the relationship between breakfast type (with or without cereal) and BMI have concluded that breakfast cereal consumers (adults and children) have lower BMIs and are less likely to be overweight than those who consume other breakfast types.

True enough, if we are talking about cereal eaters only. Kellogg's should also mention that breakfast skippers are less likely to be obese than those who eat a non-cereal breakfast, this according to Cho.

Kellogg's finally admits the existence of a key factor.

> A further explanation linking breakfast to lower body weight is that people who eat breakfast have lifestyles that promote better weight management than breakfast skippers.

Thank you. The defense rests, your Honor! But despite this insight, the brochure ends with a strong pro-breakfast statement.

> Regular consumption of breakfast plays a positive role in weight management, particularly breakfast including cereal; although a clear mechanism has yet to be defined.

The is simply erroneous. A "clear" mechanism has yet to be defined because there probably is no mechanism at all.

> Strategies and simple ideas are needed to identify barriers to breakfast eating and to encourage the consumption of a nutritious breakfast every day.

What about strategies to identify barriers to a nutritious lunch, or dinner? Not a priority, apparently.

But enough of Kellogg's. Let us move on.

Chapter 12 General Mills

On General Mills' main website, the health information provided is reasonable and not breakfast-centric.

> Our guidelines underscore the company's commitment to responsible advertising by stating that all marketing activity should respect three key steps to healthier living: balance, moderation and exercise.....If you want to lose weight, exercise more, stress-out less, and live an all-around heart-healthier lifestyle, we have some suggestions you can use throughout the day.

One of the guidelines includes exercising before breakfast, which is encouraging. So preliminary kudos to General Mills, a company that consistently leads the list of most socially responsible corporations.

More contestable claims, however, appear in General Mills subsidiary website "Eat Better America" which has on it a brochure in PDF format.

> Did you know? Cereal consumption as part of an overall healthy lifestyle may play a role in maintaining a healthy Body Mass Index (BMI) and adequate nutrient intake. Dieters who successfully maintained a weight loss of 30 pounds or more confirm that eating breakfast maximizes the likelihood of maintaining weight loss, according to National Weight Control Registry data.

Remember the National Weight Registry from the earlier chapter on Jenny Craig? The NWCR is a voluntary online database not sponsored by the U.S. Government. General Mills references the same group of weight losers that Jenny Craig did, reporting that these individuals ascribed their success to eating breakfast regularly. But from the NWRC web site itself, only 78% reported eating breakfast daily which means that 22% skip breakfast and still manage to maintain their weight loss. More importantly, not reported by General Mills was that 90% of the group reported exercising for 60 minutes a day.

Should we pull our kudos?!

Another assertion from the "Eat Better America" site.

A large study published in the Journal of the American Dietetic Association followed 2,000 American girls over a 10-year period. It found that girls who demonstrated a consistent cereal-eating pattern had healthier body weights and lower BMI than those who did not. Frequency of breakfast consumption and cereal consumption declined with age, but girls who continued to eat cereal frequently maintained a healthier body weight through adolescence.

While not specifically dealing with adults, the above summary gives the reader the distinct impression that the adolescent girls would carry over their "healthier weight" into adulthood if they just continued to eat breakfast.

The study:

Barton BA et al. *The relationship of Breakfast and cereal consumption to nutrient intake and body mass index: The National Heart, Lung and Blood Institute Growth and Health Study.* JAm Diet Assoc 2005;105:1383-1389.

From the study abstract:

Days eating breakfast were predictive of lower BMI in models that adjusted for basic demographics (ie, site, age, and race), but the independent effect of breakfast was no longer significant after parental education, energy intake, and physical activity were added to the model.

The abstract does not support the assertion in the article.

While the main focus of the PDF brochure is children, much of the content is given over to extolling the benefits of whole grains in diets for all ages — and not just for breakfast. Certainly no one will argue that cereals are not healthy foods, however the predictable catchphrases about breakfast come early on.

Breakfast is the most important meal of the day...Frequent cereal eaters tend to have healthier body weights.

The first of the two studies deals only with children and will not be discussed. The second deals with adults.

Bertrais B et al. *Contribution of ready-to-eat cereals to nutrition intakes in French adults and relations with corpulence.* Ann Nutr Metab 2000;44:249-255.

The French study looked at the eating of ready-to-eat-cereals (RTEC) and overall nutritional balance. Interestingly, it examined cereals consumed at any time of the day and not just for breakfast. The study found a positive role for RTEC whenever they were consumed and not limited to breakfast. So for adults the two General Mills' statements are not supported.

Wheaties is the first and most iconic of General Mill's ready-to-eat cereals. On the Wheaties web site the company has a promotional PDF brochure. It is written by Wheaties' "Performance Nutrition Expert" who is an exercise physiologist. The purpose is to show the reasons behind the "new" formulation of Wheaties cereal. No references are cited in it, but the author kindly sent me the eight studies which the article is based.

While the new Wheaties formulation is designed for athletes, the article makes broad assertions about the eating of breakfast and weight loss for the non-athlete.

Athletes can burn 6,000 calories a day or more, so it makes sense that Wheaties should be high in carbohydrates. The athletic body functions best on a ready supply of glucose. Carbohydrates are needed as well for a fast muscle recovery time from hard workouts, as glycogen has to be replenished.   Some statements are misleading, however, and place more importance on breakfast than is merited.

> Athletes and active individuals need a high amount of carbohydrate in their diet, and breakfast should provide a high percentage of this carbohydrate. Breakfast is unique because some of the benefits it provides have short-term or immediate effects, while other benefits are long-term. Breakfast should immediately raise the body's energy level and restore the blood glucose level to normal after an overnight fast. It should also rapidly replenish the body's carbohydrate stores. By increasing the amount of carbohydrate and using a combination of simple sugars Wheaties FUEL is very effective at providing rapid energy to get the day going with vigor and vitality, and replenishing the body's energy stores.

In the morning, as we have seen from previous chapters, the body's metabolism is doing just fine, deriving energy mainly from fats. By immediately consuming carbohydrates is more ATP going to be produced? While Wheaties suggests it will, the physiologic answer is no. The amount of ATP that can be gained from glucose is the same as the amount of ATP that can be gained from fats, as they share common aerobic pathways.

Additionally, while the morning blood sugar might be low-normal, it is still normal. The Wheaties PDF gives the impression that the body is running out of glucose, but as we have seen, glucose—essential for brain function—is being supplied as needed through the breakdown of glycogen or through gluconeogenisis, brought about by increased levels of cortisol, glucagon, and epinephrine. Also, if there is an urgent need for ATP, there is still phosphocreatine and glycogen that can be tapped. Carbohydrates will be needed eventually to replenish the glycogen and phosphocreatine, but these can be supplied later at any time during the day.

Wheaties boasts of a "balance" of simple sugars to increase performance and muscle recovery. But almost all (95%) of these sugars wind up in the serum as glucose anyway after being processed in the liver (p. 56). There is no documented advantage to one type of simple sugar over the other. Absorption might be quicker with simple sugars, but, as we have seen, the body has no immediate need for exogenous glucose in the morning.

In muscle recovery from exercise, there are more variables in play other than just glycogen replenishment. As has been suggested by the morning fast pilot study, increased growth factors, insulin, cortisol, and amino acid levels could play a greater role.

Admittedly, for the athlete the ingestion of breakfast is not an issue of concern. Athletes can eat a 500 calorie meal every two hours during the day and not gain an ounce.

The article continues:

The increased carbohydrate in Wheaties FUEL does more than simply provide a rapid and sustained supply of fuel to power the body during the morning hours. It also lowers blood cortisol levels that are at their highest in the morning.

As we have seen, the body has more than enough fuel on board to "power" through the morning. The other question concerns cortisol: are high morning levels bad for you? The physiologic answer is "no." From a common sense standpoint, the answer is also "no." This system evolved over millions of years. To say that the cortisol morning spike needs to be immediately reversed by wheat flakes must be supported by strong clinical evidence – which Wheaties does not supply.

During the night as blood glucose levels decline, cortisol is released and this stress hormone breaks down fat and protein (mainly from muscle) so that they can be converted to the energy necessary to keep us alive. If we do not consume carbohydrates and restore blood glucose during the breakfast hours, cortisol will remain elevated. If skipping breakfast becomes routine, it can have a devastating effect on the body. Chronic elevations in cortisol will result in muscle wasting and increased body fat storage, particularly in the abdominal region. It also is a strong stimulator of appetite, which can lead to unhealthy snacking during the day.

Let us review the physiologic actions of cortisol. As the body switches over to fat metabolism, cortisol is released from the adrenal cortex in response to the "stress" of a low-normal blood sugar. One of the actions of cortisol is to mobilize amino acids from protein. The amino acids are then used to make glucose (gluconeogenisis) for the primary purpose of fueling the brain cells – which function on glucose exclusively – while the rest of the body burns fats.

What Wheaties misses is that for short-term exposure, as would be the case in a morning fast or the skipping of breakfast, the protein broken down is labile protein—smooth muscle and enzymes—and not contractile protein or brain protein. Strength and athletic performance are not affected. Contractile protein is broken down only after a week of continuous exposure to high cortisol levels which occurs only in abnormal states like severe starvation or ACTH-secreting tumors (Cushing's syndrome). The same goes for abnormal fat deposition—it takes a week of continuous exposure occur. In the healthy adult, with a regular morning fast or merely skipping breakfast this is not a concern. When the stress of a morning fast, or any prolonged fast, is removed, cortisol levels fall within 30 minutes and protein and fat metabolism normalize. The protein lost to gluconeogenisis—labile or otherwise—is resynthesized.

In fact, in the short term cortisol has strong anti-inflammatory properties which are beneficial from all indications. Appetite? In the long term, over days and weeks, elevated levels of cortisol do increase appetite to high levels, but there is no problem short-term. The Cho study found that those who skipped breakfast had a lower daily caloric intake than those who ate breakfast—hunger apparently not being a problem with them.

The Wheaties article didn't mention the other stress hormones, mainly growth hormone, that increase along with cortisol. Growth hormone levels peak within 30 minutes of stimulation and then fade, but GH stimulates secondary growth factors like somatomedin C—which has a half-life of 20 hours. GH and other stress-related growth factors are essential in the making of proteins and the breakdown of fats. They are also important in muscle recovery after exercise and might play a role in mitigating affective mood disorders.

Another assertion:

> Of all the meals that we eat, breakfast is the most satiating. This satiating effect can impact food consumption for the entire day. Investigators have found that the time of day of food intake has a dramatic effect on overall daily food consumption. Eating breakfast reduces caloric intake for the entire day.

Cho, however, in his analysis of the NHAMES data — with 16,000 participants — did not find this. Also, the Rampersaud study found that breakfast-skipping adolescents consumed lower levels of calories during the day compared to their breakfast-eating counterparts.

The Wheaties PDF then veers off into the subject of breakfast and weight loss.

> Interestingly, researchers have also found that even when the same amount of calories are consumed daily that dieters who eat breakfast lose on average 50% more weight than dieters who skip breakfast. Perhaps the most compelling study on the critical role of breakfast and the ideal macronutrient combination to consume was reported in 2008. The study was conducted over eight months and compared two groups of obese women. The first four months focused on weight loss and the second four months on weight maintenance. One group consumed a low carbohydrate diet that totaled 1,085 calories per day. For this group, breakfast was the smallest meal of the day. The second group consumed a high carbohydrate diet that totaled 1,285 calories per day. For the high carbohydrate, higher calorie group, breakfast was the largest meal of the day. Conventional thinking would suggest that the group consuming the high carbohydrate, high calorie diet would lose less weight. The results were dramatic and surprising. After eight months, the low carbohydrate group

lost 10 pounds. The high carbohydrate, big breakfast group lost 37 pounds....This study reinforces the importance of breakfast, as well as the importance of consuming the appropriate macronutrients at the appropriate time to optimize function; in this case a high percentage of carbohydrate.

A win for the pro-breakfast crowd on the surface, but let us take a closer look. The reference study is from Israel:

Jakubowicz,D; Froy,O et al; *Meal timing and composition influence ghrelin levels, appetite scores and weight loss maintenance in overweight and obese adults.* Steroids 77 (2012) 323–331

The researchers divided up two groups of obese individuals, as the Wheaties article describes. Both groups had similar BMI profiles. After a four month diet protocol, both groups had lost a similar amount of weight, about 13 kilograms. When the diet ended, they were no longer on the protocol, but still saw counselors and were encouraged to continue with their diets.

In the low carbohydrate breakfast group, the weight gain was immediate, and the trend continued for four months. In the high carbohydrate breakfast group, they continued to lose weight over the four-month follow-up period.

On its face, this is good evidence for those who advocate high-carbohydrate, high-protein breakfasts. But, as has been seen with all other diet-based programs, initial losses over the years fade. A longer follow-up in this study is needed to draw any far-reaching conclusions. It would have also been very interesting for our purposes if they had a no-breakfast group for a controlled comparison.

To counter the Israeli study, Schlundt studied much the same subject years earlier in 1992.

Schlundt DG, Hill JO, Sbrocco T, Pope-Cordle J, Sharp T. *The role of breakfast in the treatment of obesity: a randomized clinical trial.* Am J Clin Nutr 1992; 55:645-651.

Briefly, this was a prospective weight loss study where the obese participants (52 women) were divided into two groups — those who ate breakfast regularly and those who skipped breakfast or ate breakfast only rarely. Both groups were assigned one of two diets, each diet containing 1200 calories per day. In one, breakfast was skipped entirely, and the calories were split over lunch and dinner. In the other, the calories were evenly split over three daily meals.

The breakfast eaters who were assigned the skip-breakfast diet lost on average almost 20 pounds at the end of the 12 week intervention, compared to just under 14 pounds that the breakfast eaters lost in the eat-breakfast group.

Not surprisingly, given the power of the myth of breakfast, Schlundt himself downplayed this his significant finding.

> Although subjects who initially ate breakfast lost more weight in the no-breakfast group, we do not believe that these individuals should be advised to stop eating breakfast because eating breakfast is associated with a reduction in total fat intake and a reduced impact of impulsive eating.

"Associated"...there's that waffle word again. Where is the causality? There is none to be found.

Take Home Points

The effect of a morning fast essentially is to drop from consuming three meals a day down to two. Common sense and 200 million years of evolution suggest that this is unlikely to be harmful to the healthy adult.

There are no scientifically rigorous studies that show a causal link between the healthy adult skipping breakfast and any adverse consequences.

Chapter 13 The Essenes and Fasting

A clinical trial involving thousands of participants and lasting for years would be the best way to prove the effectiveness of the Essene Diet morning fast and validate the pilot study. But is one really needed? A real-life study was started over 2500 years ago and lasted for more than 500 years.

The Essenes were described in detail by the Jewish historian Flavius Josephus. Josephus lived in the first century A.D. and was born only a year after Jesus' crucifixion—in the first year of Roman Emperor Caius' reign. The Essenes were also described by Philo Judaeus, who was an earlier Jewish philosopher-historian from Alexandria, Egypt.

Josephus wrote about the religious sect in his A.D. 78 opus "Wars of the Jews." Presumably, after the destruction of Jerusalem and the Second Temple in A.D. 70, the sect was outlawed by the victorious Romans—along with the Jewish High Priesthood.

The Essenes were ascetic holy men who lived communally in cities and towns in the Jewish East and who practiced a secret variant form of Judaism about which few details are known. The Essenes stand apart from the two larger orders of Jewish priests, the Pharisees and the Sadducees—both familiar to us from the New Testament.

The Sadducees have as their most famous members Caiaphas and Ananus, who were key figures in the crucifixion of Jesus.

Jesus could have been an Essene himself, though there is no hard supportive evidence for it. Certainly, Jesus at least knew of the Essenes and their philosophy for his own teachings reflect much of it.

The Essenes were physically active men by intention. They worked six days a week in the community, doing farm labor or tending livestock. Work was thought to be godly and sweating a good thing.

The Essenes were very healthy. Josephus reports that many of them lived past the century mark. As an integral part of their routine, these men would eat their first meal of the day after putting in several hours of work. According to Josephus, they would work until the fifth hour and then have their first meal.

Let us now take an extended look into the world of the Essenes. The following excerpt is taken from Josephus' *Wars of the Jews* (Whiston translation; Book II. Chapter 8).

2. For there are three philosophical sects among the Jews. The followers of the first of which are the Pharisees; of the second, the Sadducees; and the third sect, which pretends to a severer discipline, are called Essens. These last are Jews by birth, and seem to have a greater affection for one another than the other sects have. These Essens reject pleasures as an evil, but esteem continence, and the conquest over our passions, to be virtue. They neglect wedlock, but choose out other persons children, while they are pliable, and fit for learning, and esteem them to be of their kindred, and form them according to their own manners. They do not absolutely deny the fitness of marriage, and the succession of mankind thereby continued; but they guard against the lascivious behavior of women, and are

persuaded that none of them preserve their fidelity to one man.

3.These men are despisers of riches, and so very communicative as raises our admiration. Nor is there any one to be found among them who hath more than another; for it is a law among them, that those who come to them must let what they have be common to the whole order, - insomuch that among them all there is no appearance of poverty, or excess of riches, but every one's possessions are intermingled with every other's possessions; and so there is, as it were, one patrimony among all the brethren. They think that oil is a defilement; and if any one of them be anointed without his own approbation, it is wiped off his body; for they think to be sweaty is a good thing, as they do also to be clothed in white garments. They also have stewards appointed to take care of their common affairs, who every one of them have no separate business for any, but what is for the uses of them all.

4. They have no one certain city, but many of them dwell in every city; and if any of their sect come from other places, what they have lies open for them, just as if it were their own; and they go in to such as they never knew before, as if they had been ever so long acquainted with them. For which reason they carry nothing at all with them when they travel into remote parts, though still they take their weapons with them, for fear of thieves. Accordingly, there is, in every city where they live, one appointed particularly to take care of strangers, and to provide garments and other necessaries for them. But the habit and management of their bodies is such as children use who are in fear of their masters. Nor do they allow of the change of or of shoes till be first torn to pieces, or worn out by time. Nor do they either buy or sell any thing to one another; but every one of them gives what he hath to him that wanteth it, and receives from him again in lieu of it what may be convenient for himself; and although there be no requital made, they are fully allowed to take what they want of whomsoever they please.

5. And as for their piety towards God, it is very extraordinary; for before sun-rising they speak not a word about profane

matters, but put up certain prayers which they have received from their forefathers, as if they made a supplication for its rising. After this every one of them are sent away by their curators, to exercise some of those arts wherein they are skilled, in which they labor with great diligence till the fifth hour. After which they assemble themselves together again into one place; and when they have clothed themselves in white veils, they then bathe their bodies in cold water. And after this purification is over, they every one meet together in an apartment of their own, into which it is not permitted to any of another sect to enter; while they go, after a pure manner, into the dining-room, as into a certain holy temple, and quietly set themselves down; upon which the baker lays them loaves in order; the cook also brings a single plate of one sort of food, and sets it before every one of them; but a priest says grace before meat; and it is unlawful for any one to taste of the food before grace be said. The same priest, when he hath dined, says grace again after meat; and when they begin, and when they end, they praise God, as he that bestows their food upon them; after which they lay aside their [white] garments, and betake themselves to their labors again till the evening; then they return home to supper, after the same manner; and if there be any strangers there, they sit down with them. Nor is there ever any clamor or disturbance to pollute their house, but they give every one leave to speak in their turn; which silence thus kept in their house appears to foreigners like some tremendous mystery; the cause of which is that perpetual sobriety they exercise, and the same settled measure of meat and drink that is allotted them, and that such as is abundantly sufficient for them.

6. And truly, as for other things, they do nothing but according to the injunctions of their curators; only these two things are done among them at everyone's own free-will, which are to assist those that want it, and to show mercy; for they are permitted of their own accord to afford succor to such as deserve it, when they stand in need of it, and to bestow food on those that are in distress; but they cannot give any thing to their kindred without the curators. They

dispense their anger after a just manner, and restrain their passion. They are eminent for fidelity, and are the ministers of peace; whatsoever they say also is firmer than an oath; but swearing is avoided by them, and they esteem it worse than perjury for they say that he who cannot be believed without [swearing by] God is already condemned. They also take great pains in studying the writings of the ancients, and choose out of them what is most for the advantage of their soul and body; and they inquire after such roots and medicinal stones as may cure their distempers.

7. But now if any one hath a mind to come over to their sect, he is not immediately admitted, but he is prescribed the same method of living which they use for a year, while he continues excluded'; and they give him also a small hatchet, and the fore-mentioned girdle, and the white garment. And when he hath given evidence, during that time, that he can observe their continence, he approaches nearer to their way of living, and is made a partaker of the waters of purification; yet is he not even now admitted to live with them; for after this demonstration of his fortitude, his temper is tried two more years; and if he appear to be worthy, they then admit him into their society. And before he is allowed to touch their common food, he is obliged to take tremendous oaths, that, in the first place, he will exercise piety towards God, and then that he will observe justice towards men, and that he will do no harm to any one, either of his own accord, or by the command of others; that he will always hate the wicked, and be assistant to the righteous; that he will ever show fidelity to all men, and especially to those in authority, because no one obtains the government without God's assistance; and that if he be in authority, he will at no time whatever abuse his authority, nor endeavor to outshine his subjects either in his garments, or any other finery; that he will be perpetually a lover of truth, and propose to himself to reprove those that tell lies; that he will keep his hands clear from theft, and his soul from unlawful gains; and that he will neither conceal any thing from those of his own sect, nor discover any of their doctrines to others, no, not though anyone should compel him so to do

at the hazard of his life. Moreover, he swears to communicate their doctrines to no one any otherwise than as he received them himself; that he will abstain from robbery, and will equally preserve the books belonging to their sect, and the names of the angels [or messengers]. These are the oaths by which they secure their proselytes to themselves.

8. But for those that are caught in any heinous sins, they cast them out of their society; and he who is thus separated from them does often die after a miserable manner; for as he is bound by the oath he hath taken, and by the customs he hath been engaged in, he is not at liberty to partake of that food that he meets with elsewhere, but is forced to eat grass, and to famish his body with hunger, till he perish; for which reason they receive many of them again when they are at their last gasp, out of compassion to them, as thinking the miseries they have endured till they came to the very brink of death to be a sufficient punishment for the sins they had been guilty of.

9. But in the judgments they exercise they are most accurate and just, nor do they pass sentence by the votes of a court that is fewer than a hundred. And as to what is once determined by that number, it is unalterable. What they most of all honor, after God himself, is the name of their legislator [Moses], whom if any one blaspheme he is punished capitally. They also think it a good thing to obey their elders, and the major part. Accordingly, if ten of them be sitting together, no one of them will speak while the other nine are against it. They also avoid spitting in the midst of them, or on the right side. Moreover, they are stricter than any other of the Jews in resting from their labors on the seventh day; for they not only get their food ready the day before, that they may not be obliged to kindle a fire on that day, but they will not remove any vessel out of its place, nor go to stool thereon. Nay, on other days they dig a small pit, a foot deep, with a paddle (which kind of hatchet is given them when they are first admitted among them); and covering themselves round with their garment, that they may not affront the Divine rays of light, they ease themselves into that pit, after which they put the earth that was dug out again into the pit; and even this

they do only in the more lonely places, which they choose out for this purpose; and although this easement of the body be natural, yet it is a rule with them to wash themselves after it, as if it were a defilement to them.

10. Now after the time of their preparatory trial is over, they are parted into four classes; and so far are the juniors inferior to the seniors, that if the seniors should be touched by the juniors, they must wash themselves, as if they had intermixed themselves with the company of a foreigner. They are long-lived also, insomuch that many of them live above a hundred years, by means of the simplicity of their diet; nay, as I think, by means of the regular course of life they observe also. They contemn the miseries of life, and are above pain, by the generosity of their mind. And as for death, if it will be for their glory, they esteem it better than living always; and indeed our war with the Romans gave abundant evidence what great souls they had in their trials, wherein, although they were tortured and distorted, burnt and torn to pieces, and went through all kinds of instruments of torment, that they might be forced either to blaspheme their legislator, or to eat what was forbidden them, yet could they not be made to do either of them, no, nor once to flatter their tormentors, or to shed a tear; but they smiled in their very pains, and laughed those to scorn who inflicted the torments upon them, and resigned up their souls with great alacrity, as expecting to receive them again.

11. For their doctrine is this: That bodies are corruptible, and that the matter they are made of is not permanent; but that the souls are immortal, and continue for ever; and that they come out of the most subtile air, and are united to their bodies as to prisons, into which they are drawn by a certain natural enticement; but that when they are set free from the bonds of the flesh, they then, as released from a long bondage, rejoice and mount upward. And this is like the opinions of the Greeks, that good souls have their habitations beyond the ocean, in a region that is neither oppressed with storms of rain or snow, or with intense heat, but that this place is such as is refreshed by the gentle breathing of a west wind, that is

perpetually blowing from the ocean; while they allot to bad souls a dark and tempestuous den, full of never-ceasing punishments. And indeed the Greeks seem to me to have followed the same notion, when they allot the islands of the blessed to their brave men, whom they call heroes and demi-gods; and to the souls of the wicked, the region of the ungodly, in Hades, where their fables relate that certain persons, such as Sisyphus, and Tantalus, and Ixion, and Tityus, are punished; which is built on this first supposition, that souls are immortal; and thence are those exhortations to virtue and dehortations from wickedness collected; whereby good men are bettered in the conduct of their life by the hope they have of reward after their death; and whereby the vehement inclinations of bad men to vice are restrained, by the fear and expectation they are in, that although they should lie concealed in this life, they should suffer immortal punishment after their death. These are the Divine doctrines of the Essens about the soul, which lay an unavoidable bait for such as have once had a taste of their philosophy.

12. There are also those among them who undertake to foretell things to come, by reading the holy books, and using several sorts of purifications, and being perpetually conversant in the discourses of the prophets; and it is but seldom that they miss in their predictions.

13. Moreover, there is another order of Essens, who agree with the rest as to their way of living, and customs, and laws, but differ from them in the point of marriage, as thinking that by not marrying they cut off the principal part of human life, which is the prospect of succession; nay, rather, that if all men should be of the same opinion, the whole race of mankind would fail. However, they try their spouses for three years; and if they find that they have their natural purgations thrice, as trials that they are likely to be fruitful, they then actually marry them. But they do not use to accompany with their wives when they are with child, as a demonstration that they do not many out of regard to pleasure, but for the sake of posterity. Now the women go into the baths with some of

their garments on, as the men do with somewhat girded about them. And these are the customs of this order of Essens.

Specifically regarding their morning fast, the first hour of Jewish day began at 6 a.m. at daybreak. These Jewish priests likely rose before then for prayer. They worked in the morning and would take their first break at the fifth hour, or 10 a.m., when they would return to their communal house. There, the Essenes would bath, put on fresh linens, and perform rituals. It was probably near the sixth hour, or 11 a.m., when they would finally get around to eating.

After that first meal, which was taken in silence and lasted for less than half an hour, the Essenes would leave their house and return to their jobs. A second and last meal was eaten after the day's work was finished.

The Essene were considered to be an ancient sect even 2,000 years ago in Jesus' time. Flavius Josephus argues that the Greek philosopher Pythagoras patterned his cult upon the Essenes, becoming familiar with them during a sojourn on Mount Carmel in the sixth century B.C.

The Greeks and Fasting

Serious fasting and not just a delayed first meal of the day was no stranger to the ancient Greeks or most ancient societies. The Greek philosopher Pythagoras required that his potential students undergo a 40-day fast before he would teach them his philosophy. Did he adapt this from the Essenes when he studied under them?

Interestingly, this ritual could be similar to the 40 day and 40 night fast in the desert that Jesus endured, as described in the Gospel of Matthew. During the fast, Jesus was tempted by Satan.

> Then was Jesus led up of the Spirit into the wilderness to be tempted of the devil.And when he had fasted forty days and forty nights, he afterward hungered. (ASV Matthew 4:2)

Modern researchers have determined that with water the average human can survive a fast for approximately two months. Without water, death occurs within days.

Other Greek philosophers, such as Plato and Socrates, also found that fasting helped purify the mind. The Greek physician Hippocrates used fasting for therapeutic intervention in disease states.

The Egyptians

The ancient Egyptians incorporated fasting and stringent cleansing of the digestive system in their monthly routine. Herodotus, a seventh century B.C. Greek historian, writes:

> "...for three successive days each month they (the Egyptians) purge, hunting after health with emetics and clysters, and they think that all of the diseases which exist are produced in men by the food on which they live... (Histories Book II)

If the Egyptians are correct that all human disease is food based, the morning fast in the Essene Diet should have added benefits — though difficult to quantify short-term.

Fasting has been associated with spirituality and purity throughout recorded history. It makes logical sense. If one believes that men are part divine and part natural, then it follows that by denying their natural side, i.e. abstaining from food, men can better come to realize their divine essence.

Philo describes the eating habits of an Egyptian ascetic cult.

No one of them may take any meat or drink before the setting of the sun, since they judge that the work of philosophizing is one which is worthy of the light, but that the care of the necessities of the body is suitable only to darkness, on which account they appropriate the day to the one occupation, and a brief portion of the night to the other.

These ancient Egyptians fasted for 12 hours a day as a matter of course.

Ramadan

Ramadan is a Islamic religious ritual that has been practiced for more than a millennium. The devout individual is expected to fast from sunrise to sunset, much like the ancient Egyptians described by Philo. In the lunar-based Islamic Calender, the fast occurs during the entirety of the ninth month which is called Ramadan. During the fast, food and water are forbidden by day, but can be consumed at night. Physical abstinence is required as well. The purpose is to turn the heart away from earthly concerns and focus on the spiritual. Hundreds of millions of Muslims take part in this ritual every year.

In healthy adults, there have been no deleterious effects found during this ritual directly attributable to the fasting. Studies have shown that the average male loses a kilogram of weight during the month of Ramadan, but usually this is gained back within a month. One study found that during Ramadan, the lipid profiles of a cohort of young devotees actually improved.

Eat Breakfast—Lose an Empire!

If you still believe that breakfast should not be missed, this next true story from Imperial Rome might convince you otherwise.

In A.D. 37, one year after the crucifixion of Jesus, Emperor Tiberius was dying but had yet to name a successor. He knew it was time.

> But for Tiberius, upon his return to Caprein, he fell sick. At first his distemper was but gentle; but as that distemper increased upon him, he had small or no hopes of recovery. Hereupon he bid Euodus, who was that freed-man whom he most of all respected, to bring the children to him, for that he wanted to talk to them before he died. Now he had at present no sons of his own alive for Drusus, who was his only son, was dead; but Drusus's son Tiberius was still living, whose additional name was Gemellus: there was also living Caius, the son of Germanicus, who was the son of his brother [Drusus]...Tiberius... prayed to his country gods to show him a manifest signal which of those children should come to the government...so he made this to be the omen, that the government should be left to him who should come to him first the next day. When he had thus resolved within himself, he sent to his grandson's tutor, and ordered him to bring the child to him early in the morning, as supposing that God would permit him to be made emperor. But God proved opposite to his designation; for while Tiberius was thus contriving matters, and as soon as it was at all day, he bid Euodus to call in that child which should be there ready. So he went out, and found Caius before the door, for (Gemellus) was not yet come, but staid waiting for his breakfast; for Euodus knew nothing of what his lord intended; so he said to Caius, "Thy father calls thee," and then brought him in. As soon as Tiberius saw Caius.. he reflected on the power of God, and how the ability of bestowing the government on whom he would was entirely taken from him; and thence he was not

able to establish what he had intended. So (Tiberius) greatly lamented that his power of establishing what he had before contrived was taken from him, and that his grandson (Gemellus) was not only to lose the Roman empire by his fatality, but his own safety also, because his preservation would now depend upon such as would be more potent than himself...when (Caius) was settled in the government, he took off this (Gemellus)...in no long time afterward, slain by a secret plot laid against him. (Josephus *Antiquities of the Jews* Book XVIII 8-9.

Because Tiberius' nephew Caius was in attendance to him early in the morning while his own grandson, Gemellus, was away eating breakfast, Caius became the next Roman emperor. Tiberius thought it was a sign from god.

Tiberius died a few days later with Caius assuming power. History knows Emperor Caius as Caligula, the most notorious of the Caesars. Caligula executed Gemellus within year of his senate confirmation.

Certainly, this is a dark and extreme argument against breakfast, and related with tongue firmly in cheek. There is, however, a lesson to be learned here: be careful of the myths that you choose to live by for they can have unexpected consequences — and not all of them good.

Chapter 14 Living Your Life

Let us now look at the experience of one of our early participants. Joann's weight loss was not as dramatic as some, but her story illustrates the benefits of the Essene Diet and how seamlessly it can be incorporated into one's daily routine.

> Hello - I am 60 and in very good health. I do have high blood pressure that is controlled with Lisinopril (10 mg/day). I am guessing if I could take some weight off, I might be able to come off the medication. I also take an antihistamine (Singulair, 10 mg/day) for allergies, and Omeprazole (20 mg/day). I am about 200 lbs., 5'1", and have dieted since my late teens trying many variations of dieting, losing 20 lbs, gaining 20 lbs. My highest weight is what I am now. I did have my metabolism checked last summer, and it is pegged low ;-((My cholesterol is good ~180, as is my LDL and HDL. I do realize that the key to maintaining weight loss is continuing to exercise and eating right. I eat well (whole grains, lean meat, fruit, and vegetables), but I do have a sweet tooth. I am divorced with two daughters who have recently left home. I do not smoke or drink.

Joann listened to the physiology lecture explaining the program. She decided to try it. After the first several days — usually the most difficult period — Joann had this to say:

Hi. Well, a week into this, and I am down 5.4 pounds. It has been pretty easy! I have not felt hunger in the morning, and I believe it is taking less food to satisfy me. I know I need to become in tune with that, as it will make a difference. I am planning to be consistent with walking next week so I'll see how that goes.

A great report. Would she continue to lose 5 pounds a week?!

A week or so later, Joann sent another email.

I haven't lost any more weight--have been staying the same. I am easily able to stick with the diet--it doesn't seem like a "diet" ;-)) My mood is good, no cravings, and no hunger. (I am very even tempered so the whole mood question is difficult for me.) It seems I get full faster, and I feel full longer. I have started a consistent walking program so I am hoping the pounds start coming off again.

So Joann plateaued after an initial drop. She did notice, however, that her food cravings were less intrusive, and she didn't feel particularly hungry during the fast period. She was getting used to an empty stomach.

The four-week report:

Hi. I am sticking with the protocol but seem to be "stuck" at the same weight. I will go up a pound two, then back down. I started walking about 10 days ago, but that hasn't made a difference weight wise--at least not yet. I like how I feel eating this way, and I am not hungry so I will stick with it.

The lack of weight loss was disappointing, but Joann "liked" how she was feeling on the morning fast. It wasn't a diet any longer, but a natural lifestyle.

I suggested that since she was feeling so good with the five hour morning fast, that she try lengthening it for an hour or two.

Joann emailed back a week later.

Hi. I wanted to let you know that after being "stuck" at the same weight for weeks, I tried your suggestion of lengthening the mini-fast period. I lengthened it two or three times last week by an hour or two. I am happy to say that I am down another 1.2 pounds for a total of 6.4 pounds. I will keep experimenting with this and hope for continued good success. Still no real hunger or inconvenience. I am continuing to walk, and I have continued eating the same food as before but trying to be more mindful of fat content. I'm still enjoying some chocolate!

More weight was lost with her extending the fast period. If Joann is used to the sensation of an empty stomach and feels good, well, why not?

Another report came a week later.

Hi. I just wanted to let you know that things are going well for me. I have not lost additional weight, but I am sticking to the protocol. I find it very easy to stay on the program, and I feel good!

After another few weeks on the protocol, Joann still remained at the same weight level.

Hi. I am doing well. Have been sticking with the morning fast, and it is pretty much second nature to stop eating at 9 pm and not eat again until 11 am the next day. Sometimes I am able to extend the fasting time, but not always. I don't have food cravings. I took a nasty fall onto my concrete porch about a month ago (I was caring for my daughter's dog, and he lunged unexpectantly--it's a long story) so my exercise has been curtailed. Thankfully I didn't break anything or receive a concussion! I walk a little in the morning, but really haven't been able to do much. The good thing through all of this is that my weight has stayed the same. My hope is to get back to exercising soon with some vigor and extend my fasting time to see if I can drop some weight.

I had not heard from Joann for two months, and assumed that she had fallen off the protocol. I was surprised to receive a report from her a week before Christmas.

I am continuing to do well. I was sick, kind of lost my appetite and everything tasted a little off. I lost a couple more pounds and am down a total of 12 lbs. now. Continuing to eat this way has been great, and I am looking forward to getting through the holidays without a weight gain!

On Christmas day she emailed.

Hi again. I am SO EXCITED. I have lost another 2 lbs. so a total now of 14. The key for me is definitely going longer than 14 hours with the fast.

It was eight months before I heard from her again. Joann hadn't lost any more weight, but she hadn't gained any either.

I am "pretty much" sticking with the program...and have stayed at about the same weight as last fall/winter. If I go off the program and gain weight, I just go back to the program and within a few days am back to where I left off. I have found that I am easily able to stick with the program and really don't have to think about it a whole lot. It is exactly what I looked for for years in a "diet plan". I have found if I go back to my old way of eating (breakfast)...I am more hungry throughout the day, and in particular in the morning. The vicious cycle then begins.

You are right about the power of marketing. People truly believe that you should always eat breakfast and that it is unhealthy not to. It's a tough battle to fight.

Joann started the Essene Diet when she was at an all-time high weight. At 60, she was at a critical point in her life — and likely on the verge of significant and permanent weight gain.

The Essene Diet protocol, however, stopped that process cold and started her on the course of gradual weight loss. She quickly lost 5 pounds and then stabilized. At the five week mark she experimented on her own and lengthened the fast period. She lost another 2 pounds. Five months into the program, she reports losing a total of 12 pounds, largely sticking to the 14-10 track. She lost another 2 pounds on last report moving up to the 16-8 track. Joann started at 200 pounds, she is now at 186, where she is comfortable.

During this period Joann ate whatever she wanted and only exercised if she felt like it. Importantly, she likes how she feels while on the Essene Diet protocol — weight loss or no weight loss. She has lost her intrusive cravings for high-calorie sweets and eats less of them.

Joann now knows how her body works which gives her confidence. She knows that breakfast is not essential and that it is perfectly fine to live with an empty stomach. Hunger is not an issue with her anymore. The hunger impulses have been reconditioned — tamed! — through behavior modification.

Practically, Joann has learned that by extending the fast period she will lose additional weight, and she is not afraid to do so. She also knows that if she exercises more, she will also lose weight — always an option.

Joann now has all the knowledge and confidence she needs to achieve future weight loss. The only question now is how badly she wants to. It is up to her.

"Give a man a fish, and he will eat for a day. Teach a man to fish, and he will never be hungry."

An appropriate aphorism in this case.

Fine Tuning

The heart of the Essene Diet is limiting your period of food intake to 10 hours a day. The other 14 hours are dedicated to fasting, where only the drinking of water is allowed. Hydration itself is important, but drinking water also helps to stave off any hunger pangs that might otherwise develop over the first few days.

The integrity of the protocol is that for several hours a day you are forced to live with the sensation of hunger as your body metabolizes fat away. The beauty of the protocol is that you are not denied food of any type or any quantity after the fast period ends.

After a week, the perception of hunger loses its immediacy and takes a back seat to more important life concerns—as it naturally should.

The Essene Diet is easy to follow. There is no need to count calories or keep track of an exercise routine or even to check your weight. Like Terri in the first chapter, you might find that after a week or so on the diet your clothes are looser, or you are moving around better—perhaps getting into and out of cars with greater ease.

With the Essene Diet there are no counselors involved, no monthly rah-rah meetings, no pills, no supplements, no specially prepared foods. Losing weight becomes an integral part of your life and not an intrusive process that upsets it. The morning fast is taken for granted — it is how you live your life.

If you are obese (BMI>30), you can expect an early weight drop of 4-7% on the Essene Diet protocol. Those who are simply overweight (BMI 25-30) will see lower weight drops initially. After than, further weight lose will be slow and variable, as it should be. After the first few days, those on the protocol should find themselves getting full more quickly when eating during the free period — evidence of stomach shrinkage. As the days pass, hunger should cease to be an issue.

Our participants consistently reported that their cravings for high-calorie sweets diminish. One reported a drop in the urge for alcohol (!). Can the protocol have an effect on those habituated to coffee or nicotine? Remember, the brain's circuitry is constantly remodeling itself!

The protocol is flexible. The 14-10 track was patterned after the ancient Essenes, but it can be considered a baseline starting point. One of the reasons the free period ends at 9 p.m. is that I did not want participants going to bed hungry and using that as a reason to quit.

So consider the 14-10 approach a starting point. On it, you should at least not gain any more weight and your brain will have a chance to acclimatize to your stomach being empty in the morning. Tinker with the start and stop times if you wish. After a few weeks, if the rate of weight loss is not satisfactory, the fast period can easily be extended temporarily to a 16-8 or even a 18-6 track. In fact, there are plenty of people in the world who survive very well on only one meal a day. But always come back to the 14-10 track. That is your touchstone.

Experiment with diets and eating different foods during the free period if you like. And exercise regularly, of course. The test group was intentionally not encouraged to begin any new exercise programs or special diets so as not to confound the results with added variables.

Vitamin and mineral supplements were intentionally not mentioned in the science chapters. The average healthy adult who is not a vegetarian should get all the body requires in a normal diet. No harm, however, in taking them. Medications can be taken in the morning as usual — with water. For medicine that has to be taken with food, check with your doctor. It should be relatively easy to change the dosing schedule.

It goes without saying that adults with medical conditions should see their doctor first before beginning the Essene Diet protocol. Diabetics in particular, who are on drugs designed to lower their blood sugar, or anyone with endocrine problems (thyroid, adrenal) should consult their physicians.

Taking Control

If you see your physician, for any reason, you might bring up the morning fast concept and see what she or he has to say. Let us hope that your doctor doesn't raise a skeptical eyebrow and say, "Skip breakfast? Why, breakfast is the most important meal of the day!"

If that is the case, before getting another physician counter by saying that nowhere in the 12th edition of Guyton's Textbook of Medical Physiology does it say that eating breakfast is necessary.

Your physician's response should be interesting.

This brings up an important point upon which we will close. As the protocol becomes integrated into your life, as I hope it will be, prepare to deal with skeptics and naysayers. There will no doubt be a lot of them. Food and diet to many has taken on the importance of religion, and faddists will vigorously defend their beliefs. Respond to them with restraint, understanding, and...the facts.

On a grittier level, by fasting in the morning you are not only directly challenging the huge and profitable breakfast food industry but also the sizable number of companies that make billions off diet programs and weight-loss pills. And they will push back.

But don't let THEM control your life, YOU control it!

About the Author

John Hagan M.D. is a medical physician with a special interest in health issues and ancient history. Other works include *Year of the Passover* and *Fires of Rome*. Dr. Hagan lives in Minneapolis.

www.ingramcontent.com/pod-product-compliance
Lightning Source LLC
Chambersburg PA
CBHW032111280326
41933CB00009B/790